Slimming World's
best ever
recipes

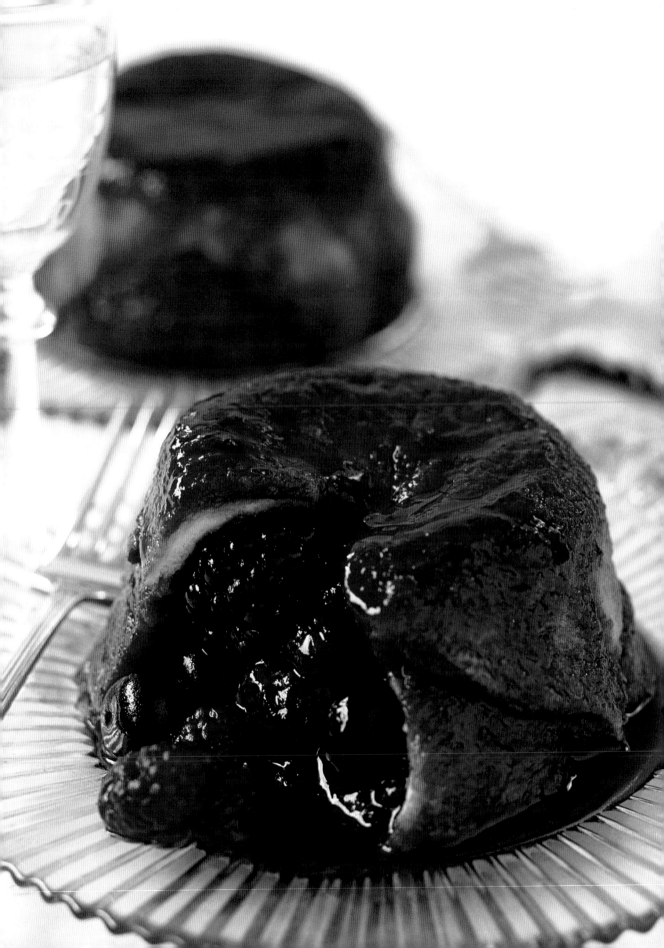

Slimming World's
best ever
recipes

40 years of Food Optimising

EBURY
PRESS

Published in 2009 by Ebury Press, an imprint of Ebury Publishing
Ebury Publishing is a division of the Random House Group

3 5 7 9 10 8 6 4

The Random House Group Limited Reg. No. 954009
Addresses for companies within the Random House Group
can be found at www.randomhouse.co.uk

A CIP catalogue record for this book is available from the British Library.

ISBN 978-0-09-192822-3

Recipes created by Sunil Vijayakar
Editor: Patricia Burgess
Designer: Nicky Barneby
Picture researcher: Victoria Hill

Food photography: Jon Whitaker
Food stylist: Sunil Vijayakar
Prop stylist: Rachel Jukes

For Slimming World
Founder and chairman: Margaret Miles-Bramwell
Managing director: Caryl Richards
Project coordinator: Beverley Farnsworth
Text by Christine Michael

The Random House Group makes every effort to ensure that the papers
used in our books are made from trees that have been legally sourced
from well-managed and credibly certified forests. Our paper procurement
policy can be found on www.randomhouse.co.uk

Printed and bound in the UK by Butler Tanner and Dennis Ltd, Frome

To buy books by your favourite authors and register for offers visit www.rbooks.co.uk

PICTURE CREDITS

The publisher would like to thank the following for providing
photographs and permission to reproduce copyright material. While every
effort has been made to trace and acknowledge all copyright holders,
we apologise should there be any errors or omissions.

Advertising Archives 190, 194, 197 (top left & bottom), 198, 200,
201, 202; Corbis 19; Getty Images 11, 17, 191, 197 (top right), 199;
Manor Photography/Alamy 192; PA Photos 195.

cookery
notes

- Both metric and imperial measures are given for the recipes. Follow either set of measures as they are not interchangeable.
- All spoon measures are level: 1 tsp = 5ml spoon, 1 tbsp = 15ml spoon.
- ⓥ Suitable for vegetarians
- ❀ Suitable for freezing
- Ovens should be preheated to the specified temperature. Grills should also be preheated.
- Use large eggs unless otherwise specified.
- Note that some of the recipes contain lightly cooked eggs. Avoid serving these to anyone who is pregnant or in a vulnerable health group, as there is a small risk of salmonella infection.
- Always use fresh herbs, unless dried herbs are suggested in the recipe.
- Use freshly ground black pepper and sea salt unless otherwise specified.

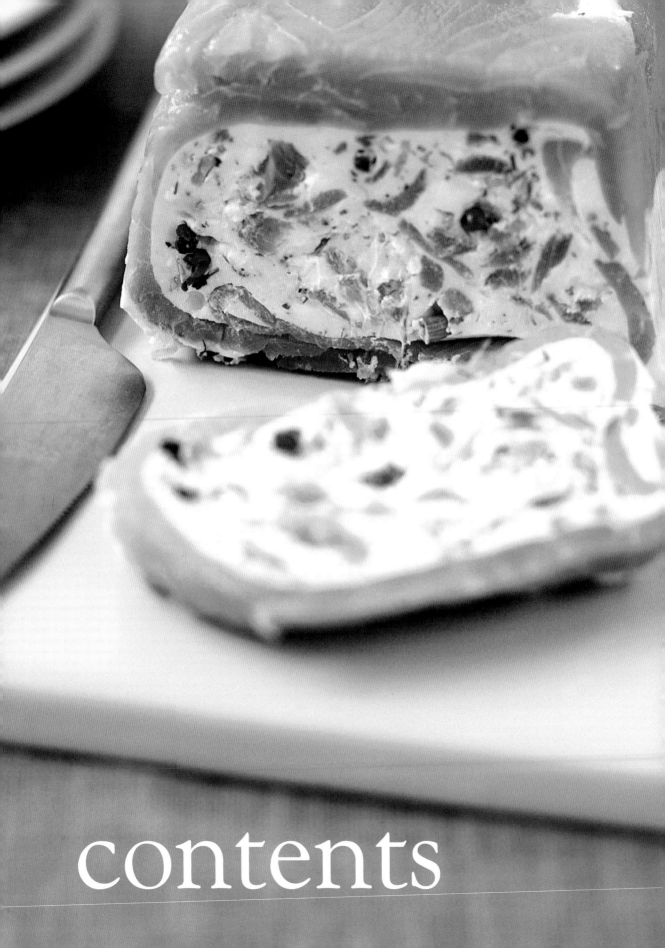

contents

foreword

Dear Reader

At Slimming World we love celebrations. We're famous for them! So imagine how we're marking our 40th birthday – 40 amazing, breathtaking, inspirational years of being able to help people conquer their weight problems for good. For me those 40 years have gone by in a blink, so I don't want a single moment of 2009 to go by without doing something really, really, extra special every single week. This glorious recipe book is a tribute to 40 years of Food Optimising recipes and to you, our readers, who deserve nothing less than the best. Welcome to the party!

When I started Slimming World in Derbyshire in 1969, I didn't even dare to dream that one day I'd be celebrating 40 amazing years as part of our huge, warm Slimming World family. It's thanks to every Slimming World member, past and present, that we've reached this milestone. Their successes have exceeded my wildest dreams!

But 40 years ago I did have dreams of creating a slimming service that was second to none. My personal experience of struggling with my weight for years, with nowhere to turn for help, fuelled me with the passion and determination to turn those dreams into reality.

Along the way it's been my immense good fortune to meet thousands of others who suffered the same diet misery that I did. I've shared with them my conviction that slimmers deserve the best eating plan, the best support and the most exceptional service we can provide. It's a terrific thrill to see our dedicated Consultants, who have all been Slimming World members themselves, delivering that service, week in and week out, to an ever-growing number of slimmers.

And 40 years on, we're dreaming of even more!

As anyone who has been involved with Slimming World in the past 40 years will tell you, we never stop questioning how we can keep improving our service to you so that it is simply the best.

That passion to give our members the best has led to many exciting innovations over the years. We developed our Green eating plan to offer a better option to slimmers who love enjoying plenty of carbohydrate-rich foods, in line with developments in nutrition science. Since then, we've extended members' choices even further with our super-flexible Mix2Max and Success Express so that everyone can Food Optimise in the way that suits them best.

We've also led the way in offering new methods of accessing our unique Slimming World service, such as our cutting-edge online BodyOptimise programme. And we're not afraid to challenge accepted wisdom, even when the easier path would be to stand back and be cautious. A dream of reaching out to the growing numbers of teenagers and young adults with weight problems led us to introduce our Family Affair programme in 2006. It's already helped over 20,000 young people to manage their weight and avoid the lifetime of ill health and unhappiness that obesity can cause.

We have also pioneered our Slimming World on Referral programme through the National Health Service. This ground-breaking scheme enables health professionals to provide the best weight-loss service available for patients, and at the time of writing we are working with over 40 Primary Care Trusts around the country.

Just after Slimming World was launched, I wrote: 'Sometimes we wish that we had a magic wand to make our members' most urgent dreams come true.' Today it is still my most heartfelt wish that we could find an instant 'cure' for weight problems. It seems, however, that all the technological 'developments' of the past 40 years have actually made life much more difficult for anyone who is prone to weight gain (and, let's face it, that's most of us!). So 40 years on, I truly believe that Slimming World has more to offer than ever before. This recipe collection, which celebrates over 100 classic dishes with a healthy Slimming World twist, gives you literally a taste of what Food Optimising has in store. We hope it whets your appetite for the complete Slimming World experience!

As you'd expect, at Slimming World we're already getting excited about the challenges of the next 40 years. But meanwhile, it's time to party – and when it comes to having fun, no one does it better than Slimming World! So come along in and join in the fun – you won't find a warmer welcome anywhere. And as thousands of Slimming World members discover every week, you'll soon have plenty of your own reasons to celebrate too!

With warmest wishes

Margaret Miles-Bramwell, FRSA
Founder and Chairman

introduction

Forty years ago the world was gathered around the television, watching something most people thought they would never see: a man walking on the moon. It was July 1969, and it felt as if the sky really was the limit.

So perhaps it's no surprise that Slimming World, launched in the same year, embodies that 'sky's-the-limit spirit'. In 2009 we're celebrating our own success story over the past 40 years: a success that has come from reaching for the stars in a different way – through our deeply felt passion for helping people reach their own full potential.

Why mark our 40 years of success with a recipe collection? Well, no Slimming World celebration would be complete without delicious food! So this book is a cook's tour of classic dishes from all over the world that have become Slimming World favourites, prepared the Slimming World way so that Food Optimisers can enjoy them to the full and still lose weight effectively and safely.

Of course, as any Slimming World member will tell you, we're about far more than food. What sets Slimming World apart, now as it did 40 years ago, is our unique approach to slimming.

In the early 1970s Slimming World's founder, Margaret Miles-Bramwell, wrote: 'Although we can generalise about people caring desperately about being overweight, nevertheless each person is different, with specific barriers to losing weight, reasons for failure up till now, particular worries, varied lifestyles. Therefore the Slimming World policy is to get to know each of our members really well and treat each of their problems individually.' Forty years ago that approach was as radical as sending a rocket into orbit!

The 1960s also saw the dawn of what parents worriedly called the 'permissive society', and this (without advocating free love or communal living!) was another spirit that Slimming World embraced from the outset.

In 2009 we're celebrating our own success story over the past 40 years: a success that has come from reaching for the stars in a different way – through our deeply felt passion for helping people reach their own full potential.

Conventional wisdom at the time was that people gained weight because they ate too much, and they ate too much because they could not control themselves. To solve the problem, the theory went, all they had to do

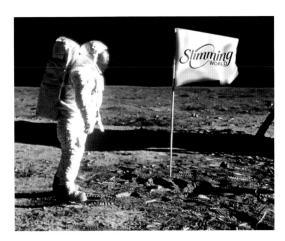

In 1969 man took his first steps on the moon – and in Derbyshire the first-ever Slimming World group was held.

was to eat less and allow themselves to be controlled by a diet sheet, a strict routine, or a 'punishment and reward' system.

The double genius of Slimming World stemmed from that deep respect for, and understanding of, individual slimmers that Margaret Miles-Bramwell wrote about so powerfully, combined with an eating plan, based on healthy, unlimited Free Foods, which freed slimmers from the burdens of hunger and guilt (see pages 12–16 for more information). The mission of the first groups Margaret set up, and of every group since, was to turn conventional wisdom about weight loss on its head and encourage each member to take control of her or his own destiny. Inviting

members to give themselves permission to eat, permission to enjoy all kinds of food, and permission to be themselves was very different from the traditional diet approach of denial and deprivation.

Along with that positive, permissive spirit and the liberating power of Free Foods, the third element Slimming World offered from the outset was flexibility. Our eating plan, Food Optimising, has stood the test of time because members have always been able to adapt it to their own lifestyle rather than the other way round.

In 1969 few people could have foreseen all the changes that our family life, diet, work, health and social life would undergo in the next 40 years. And it's probably fair to say that few people in 1969 would have predicted that Slimming World would become the market-leading, hugely influential and successful organisation it is today. And that sky's-the-limit spirit is still going strong, 40 years on! So in celebrating our anniversary, it's exciting to know that there is so much more to look forward to: we're still reaching for the stars, and the best is yet to come.

> For details of a warm and friendly group near you, call 0844 897 8000 or visit www.slimmingworld.com

40 years of Slimming World

Slimming World launched in Derbyshire in 1969 with just four groups; 40 years on we hold almost 6,000 groups every week, and are proud to be the UK's biggest and most advanced weight-management organisation. From the start, we relied on personal recommendation rather than expensive advertising campaigns to attract new members, and today word of mouth is still our most powerful recruitment tool.

So what is it about Slimming World that first brought new members through the door and delighted them so much that they couldn't wait to tell their friends and family?

Every new member, then and now, finds that at the heart of Slimming World's success is an enjoyable, effective and generous eating plan that takes an entirely fresh approach to slimming. Instead of advising you to cut portions, Slimming World offers you a long list of Free Foods – foods you can eat as much of as you like – and these aren't 'diet foods', such as lettuce or cottage cheese, but proper, filling foods, such as lean meat, fish, fresh fruit and vegetables. Instead of being given a diet sheet and strict rules about what, when and how much to eat, members swap recipes and ideas for meals, write their own menu plans and are encouraged to enjoy them whenever and wherever they want.

Then as now, members who joined Slimming World expecting to be told firmly what to do found that, in a very warm, supportive way, they were encouraged to exercise their own 'choice power' over every aspect of their weight-loss journey. Today taking control

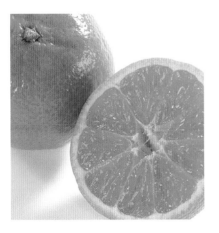
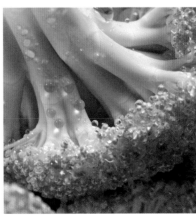
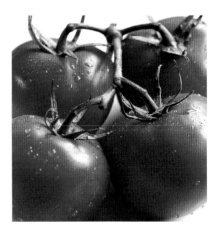

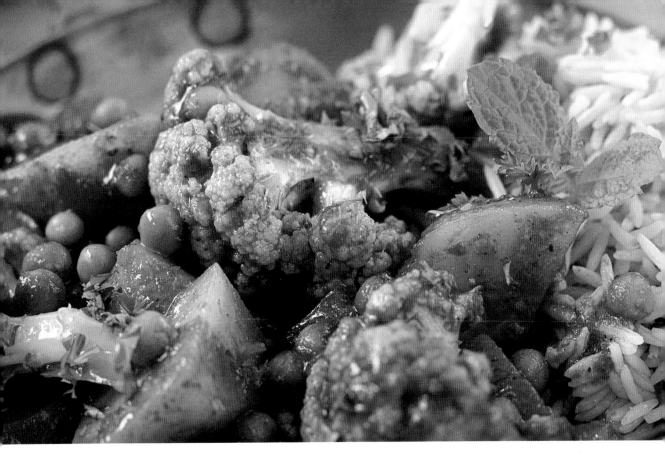

still starts from the very first meeting, when members are invited to choose their own target weight, or to decide not to set a target weight straight away if they prefer. No unreasonable targets are ever imposed.

Being invited to enjoy food again – and plenty of food at that – was a revelation to slimmers who were expecting tiny portions and 'rabbit food', just as it is today. And even those who are convinced that a diet with unlimited foods can't possibly work are amazed and thrilled to find that they lose weight even if they test Free Foods to the max.

It was all very different from the standard fare that slimmers had to endure at the time. At the start of the 1970s nutritionists knew that to lose weight, people had to expend more calories in activity than they took in as food – a fact of life that's just as true today. But they understood far less about appetite and how to satisfy it,

and the reasons why we might overeat, than we do now. Slimming diets typically involved drastic calorie cutting, and while they worked in the short term, they set slimmers up for a vicious cycle of hunger, deprivation, despair, rebellion – and more weight gain.

FOOD OPTIMISING: THE POWER OF FREE FOODS

Having suffered herself from a long-standing weight problem, Slimming World's founder Margaret Miles-Bramwell had tried many kinds of diet and become disillusioned with them all. From her own experience, she understood the misery of feeling hungry on diets with tiny portions, the shame and guilt of 'breaking the diet' and overeating, and the frustration of having to miss out on family meals and a social life because of being 'on a diet'. And as an intelligent, adult woman, she resented being

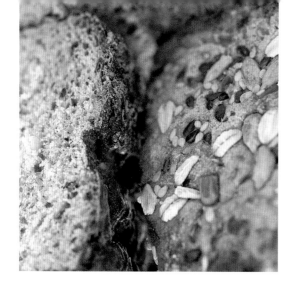

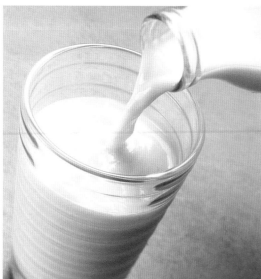

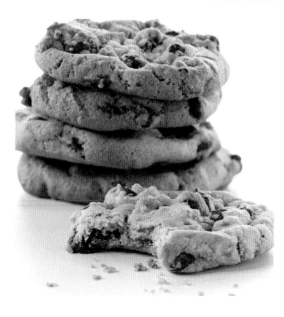

made to feel like a naughty schoolgirl if she broke the rules.

So Slimming World started with a new philosophy: to empower slimmers to feel free around food and to eat as 'normal' people do, without counting or feeling guilty about every mouthful. This way of eating, which has been Slimming World's approach since day one, is now a highly sophisticated yet very easy-to-follow system called Food Optimising.

By basing their meals on Free Foods, Slimming World members can eat without ever going hungry, and still lose weight every week. Free Foods include healthy, everyday basics, such as pasta, rice, potatoes, eggs, lean meat, chicken and fish, plus fruit and vegetables – a hugely flexible list that can accommodate every lifestyle, every occasion and everyone's food likes and dislikes.

How can you eat as much of these as you like and lose weight? The answer lies in the science of appetite satisfaction: Free Foods are high in either protein or carbohydrate, the two food groups that are known to be the most satisfying to the appetite and that help us feel fuller for longer. Yet because Free Foods are low in fat and sugar, and some are high in fibre, they are also relatively low in calories compared to other foods. Free Foods are the way that Slimming World members can pile their plates with confidence, even when people comment, 'I thought you were on a diet!'

There's even more to Food Optimising than Free Foods. The second element of the eating plan is Healthy Extras: foods such as cheese, dairy products, wholemeal bread, cereals and dried fruit. Healthy Extras are important because they are either high in fibre or rich in minerals, all of which are essential for a healthy diet. Food Optimisers choose up to four measured servings of these every day in addition to unlimited Free Foods. No wonder many members say they are eating more than ever before and still losing weight!

One crucial part of Food Optimising's philosophy is that no foods are banned and that all foods can be enjoyed, so Food Optimisers are encouraged to enjoy an allowance of foods that have a 'Syn value' every single day. 'Syn' stands for 'synergy' – the power of different elements to work together to create an even more powerful result. Syns are the way that Food Optimisers can relax and enjoy a daily bar of chocolate, a packet of crisps, a creamy sauce with dinner,

or a glass of wine if they wish. Many slimmers find that Syns make all the difference between feeling that they are 'on a diet' and have to give up their favourite foods, and being confident that they have found a healthy way of eating they can stick to for life.

In fact, Food Optimising is so healthy that it can safely be followed by pregnant women and breastfeeding mums (with their midwife's approval). Many women every year find, to their huge relief, that Food Optimising helps them maintain their weight for a healthy pregnancy and regain a healthy weight afterwards, while ensuring that their baby enjoys the best possible start in life.

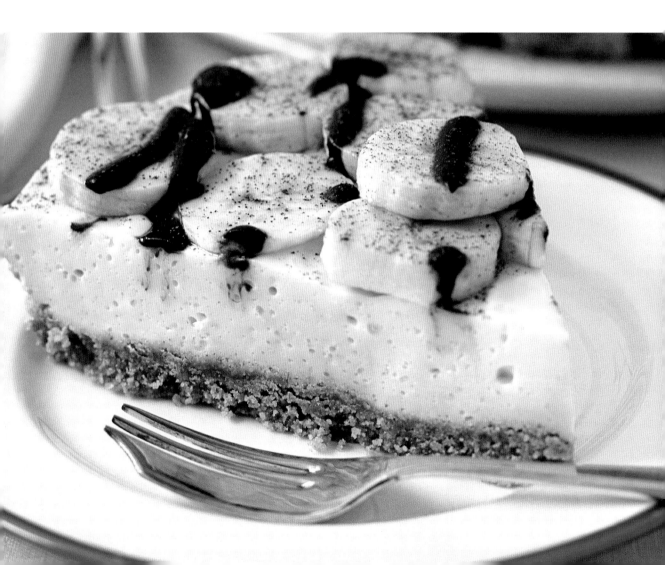

- **Original choice:** Food Optimising's Original choice is for you if your absolute favourites are roast beef and all the trimmings, a mixed grill or a cooked breakfast. Lean, satisfying, protein-rich foods, including beef, chicken, lamb, bacon, turkey, fish and seafood, are all Free on the Original choice, as well as all fresh fruit and nearly all vegetables, eggs and dairy products, such as very low fat natural yogurt and fromage frais. Add daily servings of Healthy Extras, such as wholemeal bread, potatoes, high-fibre breakfast cereals and cheese or milk, to provide even more energy, fibre, vitamins and minerals, then decide how to use your Syns for the day.

- **Green choice:** Do you just love tucking into meals such as a huge jacket potato with beans, a plate of delicious pasta, or a veggie curry with plenty of rice? Then you'll love Food Optimising's Green choice. Even on the hungriest days, satisfy your appetite with carbohydrate-rich comfort foods, such as potatoes, pasta, rice, couscous and pulses – all are Free Foods on Green – along with all fresh fruit and vegetables, eggs and some dairy products, such as very low fat natural yogurt and fromage frais. Add delicious daily Healthy Extras, such as lean meat or fish, wholemeal bread, high-fibre cereals and cheese or milk, to supply even more fibre, vitamins and minerals, then add in your daily Syns – if you can possibly find room, that is!

- **Mix2Max:** This gives you the option to go Green or Original at each meal – perfect if you aren't able to plan too far ahead, or just prefer to see what you fancy at the time. So if you'd like hash browns and beans for breakfast, grilled salmon for lunch, and a big vegetable chilli and rice for supper – go right ahead! You still get to choose Healthy Extras and Syns every day, so Mix2Max is just as healthy, satisfying and enjoyable as Green and Original. And it's even more flexible, so once you're happy with how the Green and Original choices work for you, Mix2Max can be a really useful extra option for days when you're eating on the move or find that life gets in the way of your dinner plans.

- **Success Express:** We all have times when we'd like to kick-start our weight loss a bit without resorting to extremes, such as missing meals (as if!) or living on lettuce. This is where Success Express comes in: it's the Food Optimising choice for the times when you want to focus on results without ever going hungry. Success Express meals are based on Superfree Foods (which are Free on Green *and* Original) and Free Foods, and there's no weighing or measuring, as you fill your plate on a two-thirds Superfree, one-third Free principle. It's a more specialist choice than Green or Original because it works slightly differently, but as you'd expect from Food Optimising, it's enjoyable, flexible and generous too. Members familiar with the Green and Original choices report that Success Express lives up to its name.

- **Free2Go:** This plan makes healthy eating easy and enjoyable for young people aged 11–15, allowing them to manage their weight, enjoy their favourite foods and lead their social life without worrying about the 'diet' issue. With Free2Go, Food Optimisers fill up on unlimited Green *and* Original Free Foods (without worrying which day they're on), a long list of Healthy Extra choices, most in unlimited quantities, and steadily reduce the number of high-fat or high-sugar foods they eat each day. The emphasis is on making 'cool swaps' towards healthier foods.

GROUP SUPPORT: THE HEART OF SLIMMING WORLD

From the outset, Margaret Miles-Bramwell was determined that there was one other thing, apart from hunger, that Slimming World members should never have to experience – humiliation.

The idea that each member should enjoy the respect and understanding of the rest of the group and their Consultant, who was there to encourage and support, not to instruct or to patronise, was truly radical at the start of the 1970s, when being overweight was seen as a sign of greed, laziness, or both.

Margaret knew only too well that the biggest problem for slimmers is often not their weight, but the burden of low self-esteem coupled with a lack of faith in their own abilities – both of which they bring with them to the group. So since those early days, new members joining Slimming World find the room set up not like school with chairs in rows, but in a horseshoe shape so that everyone can contribute if they want to. And in IMAGE Therapy (it stands for Individual Motivation and Group Experience) they find that they're encouraged to share their successes, give and receive compliments, ask for and offer suggestions, and to think about what they want to achieve and what might hold them back. Best of all, laughter and fun are essential parts of the Slimming World mix – it's a great night out! Members whose weight loss is going well leave their meeting on an unbeatable high, while those who are struggling

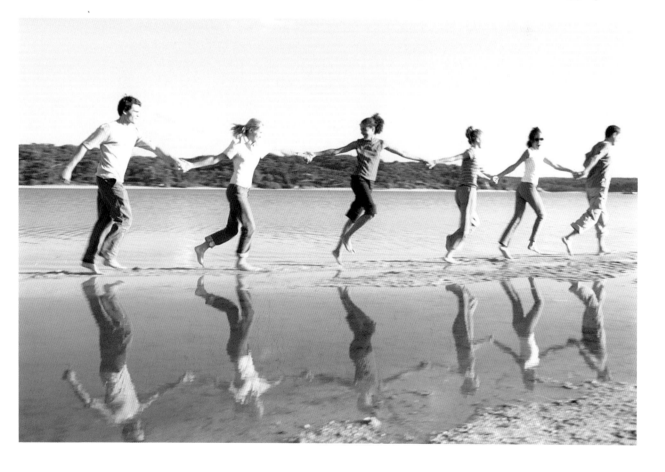

feel that they have the support of the whole group and have a warm glow to see them through the week ahead.

The spirit of sharing and support continues between meetings too; a buddy system called Lifelines – originally by telephone, now just as often by text or email – keeps members in touch with each other, and for the past ten years Slimming World group members have had *free* access to the Slimming World website. The most important thing is that members know they are assured of a warm welcome at their group no matter what. It can be hard enough to join a slimming club in the first place; coming back when you know you haven't had a good week is harder still. But when they do, members can expect praise and applause as the rest of the group know it has taken courage to return.

Achieving this balance of motivation, support, humour and respect doesn't come about by accident. Slimming World's 2,500 Consultants, who have all been members themselves, are highly trained in techniques to help them empathise with others, motivate them to achieve, and raise their awareness of issues that might be preventing them from reaching their goals.

BODY MAGIC: FIT FOR LIFE

When Slimming World launched, the emphasis in groups was focused on the eating plan and offering support to reach goals; members were encouraged to exercise, but there was no formal programme in place. That's all changed in the past few years with the introduction of Body Magic, a system of motivating members to be active that complements Food Optimising and IMAGE Therapy in its power to speed weight loss and boost confidence. Here again, Slimming World took advantage of the most

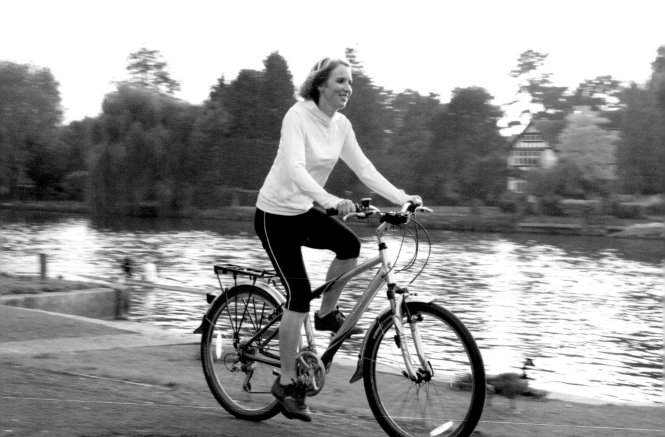

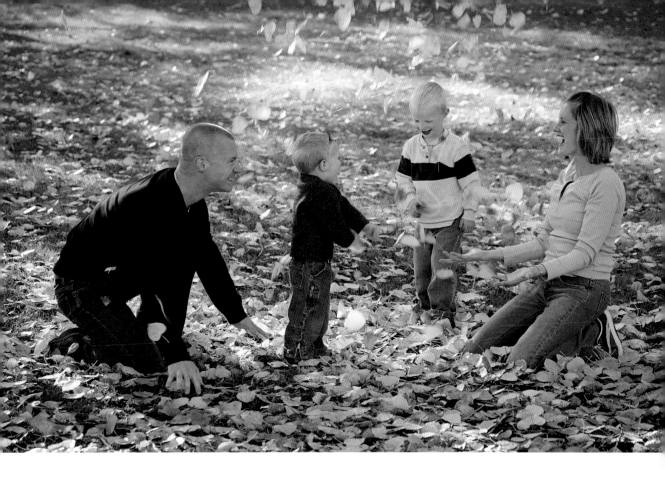

up-to-date thinking on exercise, which has moved on since the days of 'no pain, no gain' in the 1980s and '90s.

Evidence now suggests that building activity into everyday life is more effective than intense bursts of exercise at the gym or out running. Every extra bit of activity, whether it's walking to the shops or taking the stairs instead of the lift, can help to improve fitness and expend energy.

In any event, after spending so long encouraging personal choice, the last thing you'd expect from Slimming World is a rigid exercise plan! So just as Food Optimising offers you the opportunity to improve your relationship with food, so Body Magic invites you to do the same with exercise. Body Magic isn't compulsory, but members who take part, starting from their current level of activity, can achieve recognition and gain awards for every extra block they build into their lives, such as

making time for a brisk walk, going for a swim, or having a kickabout in the park.

A POWERFUL COMBINATION

Forty years ago few people could have foreseen just how big a problem obesity would become. In the chapters on pages 189–202 we look at how our changing lifestyle has had a dramatic impact on our weight and health, and how our environment has made it harder than ever to maintain a healthy weight. In today's 'obesogenic' world there has never been a greater need for an effective, practical method of weight management. The powerful combination of Food Optimising, group support and lifestyle-based activity puts Slimming World at the forefront of weight management in the UK – and it's the reason why so many thousands of people every week achieve the weight loss they've always dreamed of.

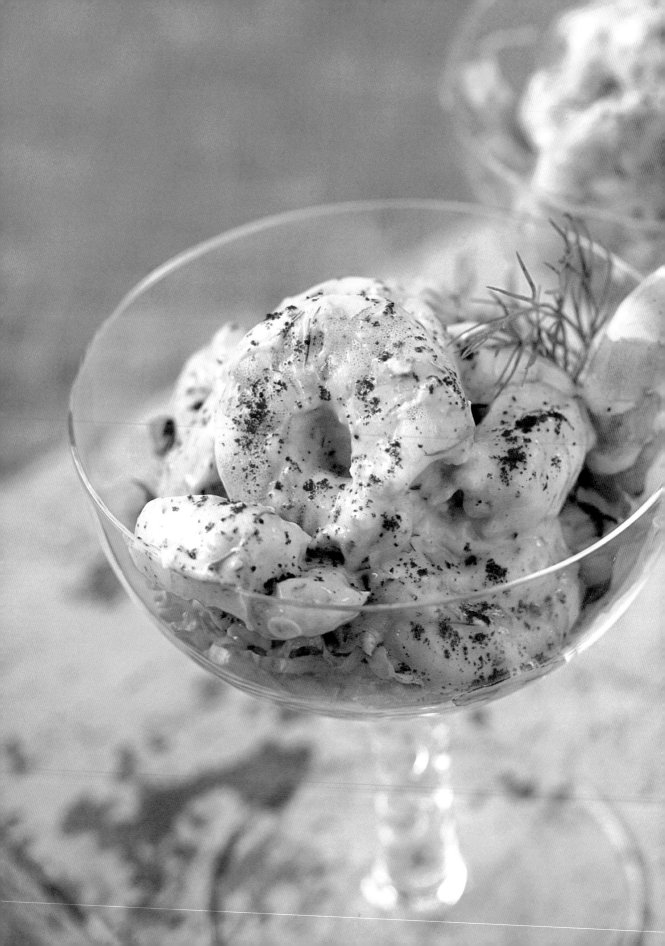

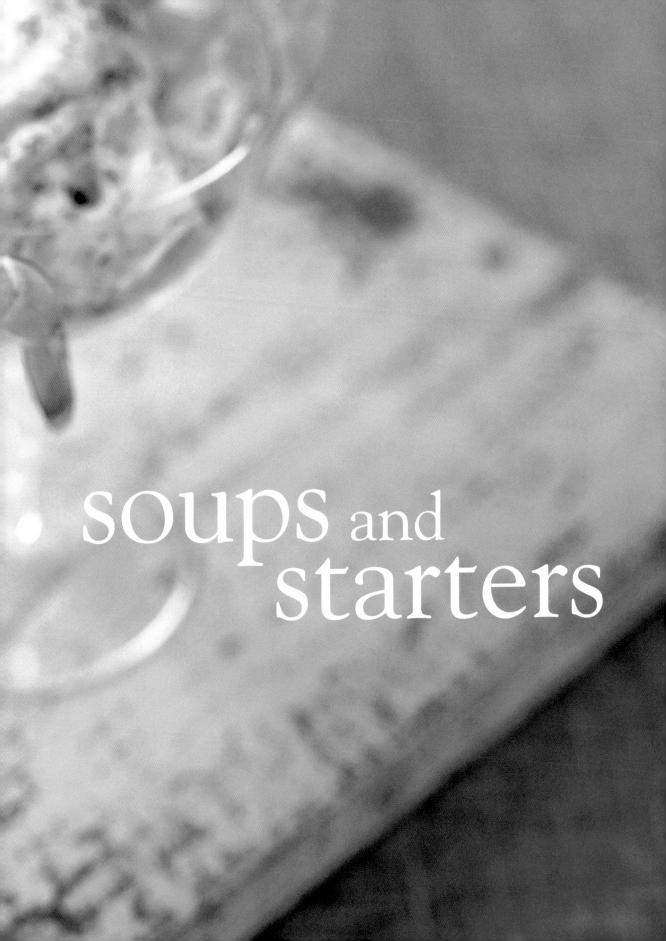

soups and starters

watercress
soup

Packed with goodness and flavour, this peppery soup looks amazing and is sure to warm you up on a cold winter's day.

SERVES 4 Ⓥ ❋
EASY
Syns per serving
Green: Free
Original: 1½

Preparation time 10–12 minutes
Cooking time about 15 minutes

2 onions, peeled and finely chopped

2 garlic cloves, peeled and finely chopped

1 large potato, peeled and cut into 1cm/½in dice

200g/7oz watercress, finely chopped

1 litre/1¾ pints water or stock made with Vecon

6 tbsp finely chopped parsley

salt and freshly ground black pepper

To serve

very low fat yogurt

watercress sprigs

1. Place the onions, garlic, potato, watercress, water or stock and parsley in non-stick saucepan over a medium heat and bring to the boil. Cover and cook gently for 10–12 minutes, or until the potatoes are tender. Season well.

2. Using a hand-held blender or food processor, blend the soup until smooth. Ladle into warmed bowls and serve with a swirl of yogurt and a sprig of watercress.

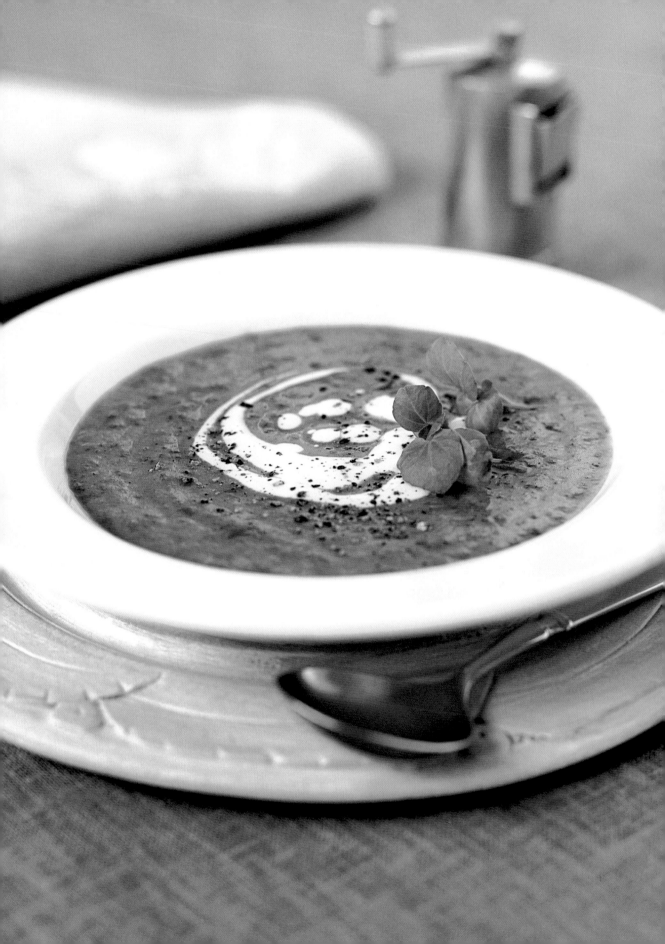

leek
and potato soup

Quick and easy quick to make, this soup uses everyday ingredients to great effect. If it's not already a favourite, it soon will be.

SERVES 4 Ⓥ ❋
EASY
Syns per serving
Green: Free
Original: 3½

Preparation time 6–8 minutes
Cooking time about 15 minutes

4 leeks, white parts only, very thinly sliced

2 garlic cloves, peeled and finely chopped

2 large potatoes, peeled and cut into 1cm/½in dice

1 litre/1¾ pints water or stock made with Vecon

salt and freshly ground black pepper

4 tbsp very finely chopped chives

To serve
very low fat natural yogurt

1. Place the vegetables and water or stock in a non-stick saucepan over a medium heat and bring to the boil. Cover and cook gently for 10–12 minutes, or until the potatoes are tender. Season well.

2. Using a hand-held blender or food processor, blend the soup until smooth. Stir in the chives, then ladle the soup into warmed bowls and top with a swirl of yogurt.

pea and mint soup

Although this is a summer classic, it can be enjoyed at any time of year.
The beautiful pale green colour and smooth texture with a hint of garlic
make a really delicious combination.

SERVES 4 Ⓥ ❄

EASY

Syns per serving
Green: Free
Original: 5½

Preparation time 15 minutes
Cooking time under 25 minutes

1 onion, peeled and finely
chopped

2 sticks celery, finely chopped

2 garlic cloves, peeled and
finely chopped

600g/1lb 6oz frozen peas

1 litre/1¾ pints water or stock
made with Vecon

6 tbsp very finely chopped
mint

To serve
very low fat natural yogurt
mint leaves

1. Place the onion, celery, garlic, peas and water or stock in a non-stick saucepan over a medium heat and bring to the boil. Reduce the heat to medium and cook for 20 minutes.

2. Using a hand-held blender or food processor, blend the soup with the chopped mint until smooth. Remove from the heat and serve immediately, drizzled with the yogurt and garnished with mint leaves.

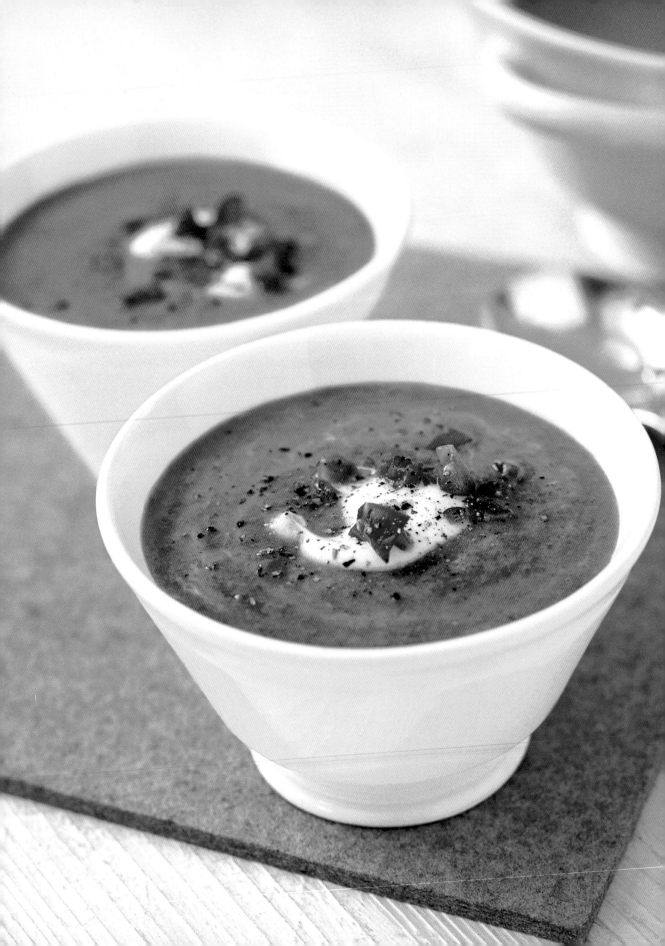

classic
tomato soup

This familiar and comforting soup is ideal for an autumn or winter lunch, and can be served with a green salad.

SERVES 4 Ⓥ ❄
EASY
Syns per serving
Original: Free
Green: Free

Preparation time 10 minutes
Cooking time under 25 minutes

Fry Light

1 onion, peeled and finely chopped

2 sticks celery, finely chopped

2 garlic cloves, peeled and finely chopped

1 carrot, peeled and finely diced

1 litre/1¾ pints water or stock made with Vecon

1 x 400g can chopped tomatoes with herbs

1 tsp artificial sweetener

salt and freshly ground black pepper

200g/7oz very low fat natural fromage frais

To serve

very low fat natural fromage frais

finely chopped tomatoes

1. Spray a saucepan with Fry Light and place over a medium heat. Add the onion, celery, garlic and carrot and stir-fry for 2–3 minutes.

2. Add the water or stock, tomatoes and sweetener and bring to the boil. Reduce the heat to medium and cook for 15–20 minutes. Remove from the heat, season well and, using a hand-held blender or food processor, blend until smooth. Return the soup to the pan and stir in the fromage frais.

3. Ladle the soup into warmed bowls and serve immediately, garnished with a little fromage frais and chopped tomatoes.

french
onion soup

Slow-cooking the onions and garlic gives a distinctive caramelised
sweetness to the flavour of this soup – a real taste of France.

SERVES 4 Ⓥ ❋
EASY
Syns per serving
Original: Free
Green: Free

Preparation time 15 minutes
Cooking time about 35–40
minutes

Fry Light

6 medium onions, peeled and
thinly sliced

1 garlic clove, peeled and
thinly sliced

1 tbsp thyme leaves

1 litre/1¾ pints water or stock
made with Vecon

salt and freshly ground black
pepper

To serve

freshly chopped parsley

1. Spray a heavy-based saucepan with Fry Light. Add the onions
   and garlic and sauté for 20–25 minutes over a very low heat,
   until golden brown.

2. Add the thyme and water or stock, bring to the boil and simmer
   for about 10 minutes. Season the soup, scatter with the parsley
   and serve immediately.

creamy mushroom soup

A hearty, traditional soup, just like Mum used to make! The mushrooms and potatoes combine to create a smooth, creamy texture.

SERVES 4 ⓥ ❋

EASY

Syns per serving
Green: Free
Original: 1½

Preparation time 20 minutes
Cooking time under 30 minutes

Fry Light

2 onions, peeled and finely chopped

2 garlic cloves, peeled and finely chopped

1 large potato, peeled and cut into 1cm/½in dice

500g/1lb 2oz button or chestnut mushrooms, finely chopped

1.5 litres/2½ pints water or stock made with Vecon

salt and freshly ground black pepper

6 tbsp very finely chopped parsley

200g/7oz very low fat natural fromage frais

To serve
very low fat natural fromage frais

1. Spray a non-stick saucepan with Fry Light and place over a medium heat. Add the onions, garlic, potato and mushrooms and stir-fry over a high heat for 5–6 minutes.

2. Add the water or stock and bring to the boil. Cover and cook gently for 15–20 minutes, or until the vegetables are tender. Season well.

3. Remove from the heat and stir in the parsley and fromage frais. Using a hand-held blender or food processor, blend the liquid until smooth. Ladle the soup into warmed bowls and serve with a dollop of fromage frais.

asparagus
with hollandaise sauce

You could serve this very tasty and simple starter as an accompaniment to grilled or poached salmon for an Original day meal.

SERVES 4 ⓥ

EASY

Syns per serving
Original: 1
Green: 1

Preparation time 10 minutes
Cooking time 10–12 minutes

800g/1lb 12oz asparagus spears

For the hollandaise sauce

6 tbsp extra light mayonnaise

200g/7oz very low fat natural fromage frais

juice and finely grated zest of 1 large lemon

75ml/3fl oz warm water or stock made with Vecon

salt and freshly ground black pepper

1. Trim the base of the asparagus spears and, using a vegetable peeler, lightly peel away the skin from the bottom half of each spear. Place the asparagus in a large pan of lightly salted boiling water and cook for 8–10 minutes, or until just tender. Drain thoroughly.

2. While the asparagus is cooking, place all the sauce ingredients in a blender and process until smooth. Season well.

3. To serve, divide the asparagus between warmed plates and spoon the sauce over the top.

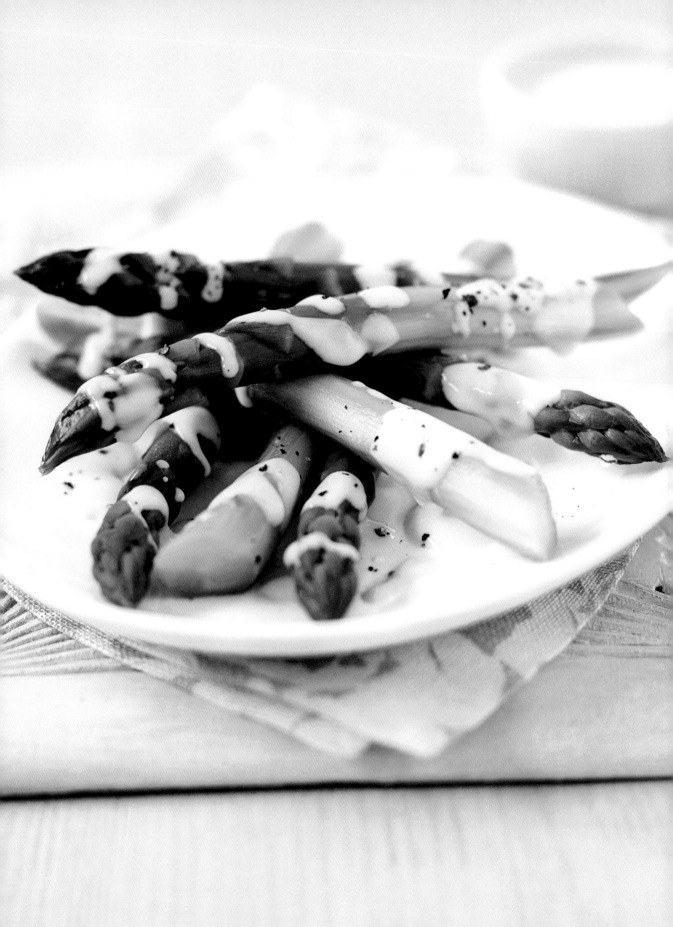

stuffed garlic and spinach
mushrooms

The classic stuffing of garlic and spinach with a hint of nutmeg brings out the woody flavour of these grilled mushrooms.

SERVES 4 Ⓥ

WORTH THE EFFORT

Syns per serving
Original: 6
Green : 6

Preparation time 5 minutes
Cooking time about 20 minutes

8 large flat field mushrooms, cleaned
Fry Light
salt and freshly ground black pepper
4 garlic cloves, peeled and crushed
150g/5oz cooked spinach, finely chopped
a pinch of grated nutmeg
110g/4oz Parmesan cheese, grated

1. Preheat the grill to medium hot. Finely chop the mushroom stalks and set aside. Spray the mushroom caps all over with Fry Light and place on a grill rack, gill-side up. Grill gently for 5–6 minutes, then turn them over, season well and grill for another 5 minutes, or until they start weeping black juice. Turn them over so that they are gill-side up again and set aside until needed.

2. Spray a large, non-stick frying pan with Fry Light and place over a high heat. Add the garlic, spinach and reserved chopped mushroom stalks, stir-fry for 4–5 minutes, then add the nutmeg.

3. Preheat the grill until hot. Season the spinach mixture and divide between the mushrooms. Sprinkle over the Parmesan and place under the grill for 2–3 minutes, or until the cheese has melted. Serve immediately.

cheesy baked potato skins
with creamy herbed dip

This wonderful starter also makes a terrific snack for the family while watching TV. It's a healthy alternative to crisps or crackers, and will disappear in a flash.

SERVES 4 Ⓥ

WORTH THE EFFORT

Syns per serving

Green: 4

Original: 6

Preparation time 20 minutes

Cooking time about 30 minutes

4 large potatoes, unpeeled and cut into wedges

6 spring onions, finely chopped

6 ripe plum tomatoes, finely chopped

1 tsp dried mixed herbs

110g/4oz reduced fat Cheddar cheese, roughly grated

For the dip

400g/14oz very low fat natural fromage frais

1 garlic clove, peeled and finely grated

finely grated zest of 1 lemon

6 tbsp finely chopped mixed herbs (chives, dill and parsley)

salt and freshly ground black pepper

1. Start by making the dip. Mix together the fromage frais, garlic, lemon zest and herbs. Season well and chill until needed.

2. Preheat the oven to 220°C/Gas 7. Place the potatoes in a large saucepan of lightly salted boiling water and cook for 3–4 minutes. Drain thoroughly and, when cool, scoop out the flesh from each wedge, leaving a 1cm/½in thickness next to the skin (save the scooped-out potato for mash or another recipe). Place the potatoes, flesh-side up, on a baking sheet lined with non-stick baking parchment.

3. Combine the spring onions, tomatoes and dried herbs in a bowl and season well. Spoon the mixture into the potato wedges, top with the cheese and bake in the oven for 20–25 minutes, or until crisp and golden. Serve immediately with the dip.

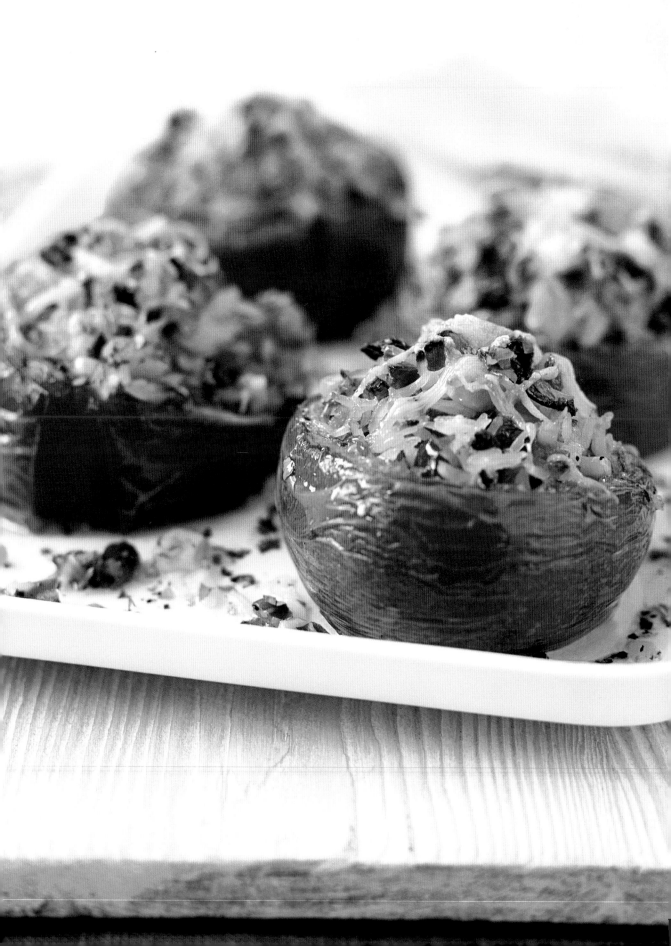

stuffed
tomatoes

Here's a great way to use up any leftover rice. The filled tomatoes not only look impressive, but taste delicious too – the perfect starter.

SERVES 4 Ⓥ

WORTH THE EFFORT

Syns per serving

Green: 4

Original: 11

Preparation time 20 minutes

Cooking time under 30 minutes

4 very large beefsteak
tomatoes

salt and freshly ground black
pepper

Fry Light

1 small red onion, peeled and
finely diced

110g/4oz green beans,
trimmed and cut into 1cm/½in
lengths

1 carrot, peeled and cut into
1cm/½in dice

110g/4oz canned sweetcorn
kernels

½ red pepper, deseeded and
very finely diced

100ml/3½fl oz water or stock
made with Vecon

300g/11oz cooked long grain
rice

110g/4oz reduced fat Cheddar
cheese, grated

To serve

freshly chopped parsley

1. Preheat the oven to 220°C/Gas 7. Cover a chopping board with kitchen paper.

2. Slice the tops off the tomatoes and scoop out the flesh and seeds. Season the insides of the tomatoes and place, cut-side down, on the prepared board. Set aside.

3. Spray a large, non-stick frying pan with Fry Light and place over a medium heat. Add the onion, beans, carrot, sweetcorn and red pepper and stir-fry for 3–4 minutes. Add the water or stock and bring to the boil over a high heat. Reduce the heat and cook, stirring, for 3–4 minutes.

4. Add the rice to the pan and mix well. Cook for 3–4 minutes, until the mixture is piping hot. Season well and remove from the heat.

5. Place the tomatoes, cut-side up, on a baking sheet and fill with the rice mixture. Sprinkle over the cheese and place in the oven for 12–15 minutes. Scatter the parsley over the top of the tomatoes and serve immediately.

waldorf
salad

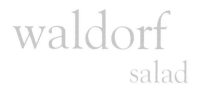

Named after the famous New York hotel where it was originally created, this salad combines sweet and savoury ingredients in a tangy dressing. Serve it as a refreshing starter, or as an accompaniment to grilled chicken.

SERVES 4 ⓥ

EASY

Syns per serving
Original: 3
Green: 3

Preparation time 20–25 minutes

1 medium celeriac

juice of 1 lemon

4 russet apples, peeled and cored

4 sticks celery, finely sliced

For the dressing

150g/5oz extra light mayonnaise

2 tsp white wine vinegar

1 tsp Dijon mustard

a pinch of artificial sweetener

salt and freshly ground black pepper

To serve

15g/½oz chopped walnuts

1. Start by making the dressing. Place the mayonnaise, vinegar, mustard and sweetener in a bowl and mix well. Season to taste and set aside.

2. Peel the celeriac and cut into large, manageable chunks. Using a mandolin, pare the celeriac pieces into thin strips. Place them immediately in a large bowl with the lemon juice and just enough water to cover. Stir well.

3. Prepare the apples in exactly the same way as the celeriac.

4. Drain the apples and celeriac and toss them in the dressing. Season to taste and pile into the centre of a large serving bowl. Scatter the walnuts over and serve.

houmous

with vegetable crudités

While versions of this popular Middle Eastern dip can be found in practically every supermarket, this is a delicious low-Syn alternative, which makes a great starter or snack.

SERVES 4 Ⓥ
EASY
Syns per serving
Green: 1
Original: 9

Preparation time 15 minutes
plus chilling

500g/1lb 2oz canned
chickpeas, rinsed and drained

juice of 1 lemon

4 garlic cloves, peeled

1 tbsp tahini paste

1 tsp paprika

3 tbsp chopped flat-leaf
parsley

3 tbsp chopped coriander

3 tbsp chopped mint

250g/9oz very low fat natural
yogurt

To serve

vegetable crudités (carrot,
celery, cucumber, radish, red
pepper, etc.)

1. Place the chickpeas in a food processor and blend until coarsely chopped. Add the remaining ingredients and process until fairly smooth. Transfer the mixture to a serving bowl and chill until needed.

2. To serve, place the houmous bowl in the centre of a large platter and surround with the crudités of your choice.

eggs benedict

This classic brunch dish of poached eggs served on wilted spinach leaves with slices of ham makes an indulgent start to a lazy Sunday.

SERVES 4

EASY

Syns per serving
Original: 3
Green: 5

Preparation time 10 minutes
Cooking time about 10 minutes

Fry Light

300g/11oz baby spinach leaves

1 garlic clove, peeled and crushed (optional)

salt and freshly ground black pepper

8 tbsp very low fat natural fromage frais

¼ tsp mustard

1 tbsp finely chopped tarragon

1 tbsp finely chopped parsley

2 x 50g/2oz wholemeal rolls, halved and toasted

4 x 25g/1oz slices lean ham

4 poached eggs

1. Spray a large, non-stick frying pan with Fry Light and place over a medium heat. Add the spinach and garlic, if using, and stir-fry until the spinach has wilted. Season well and keep warm.

2. In a small saucepan gently heat the fromage frais, mustard and chopped herbs, whisking all the time until warm (take care not to let it boil). Remove, season well and keep warm.

3. To assemble, place each toasted roll half on a serving plate, cut-side up, and cover with a slice of ham. Divide the spinach mixture between the rolls and top each with a poached egg. Spoon over the sauce and serve immediately.

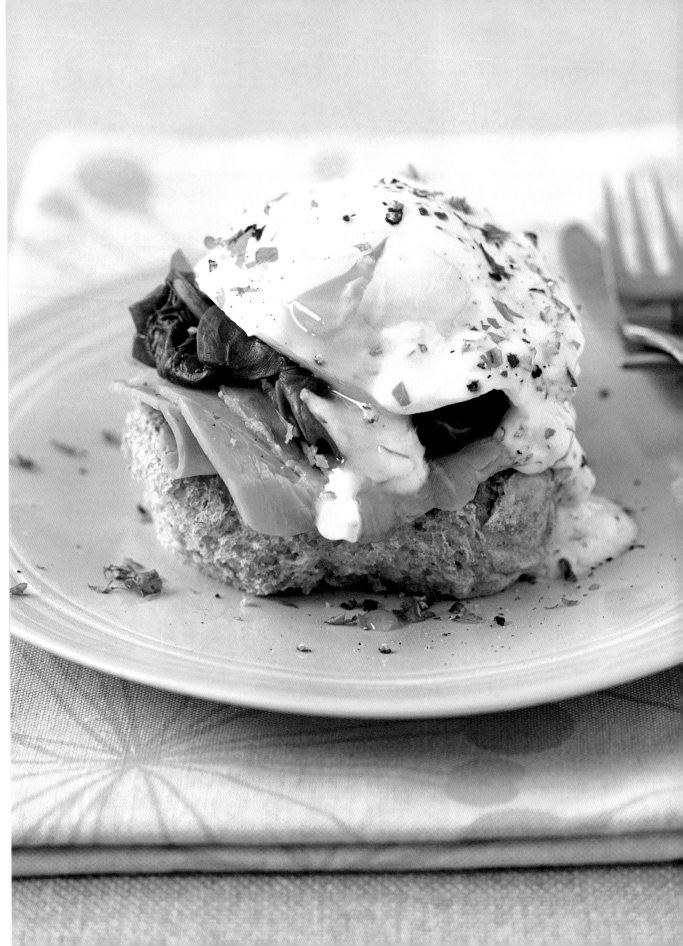

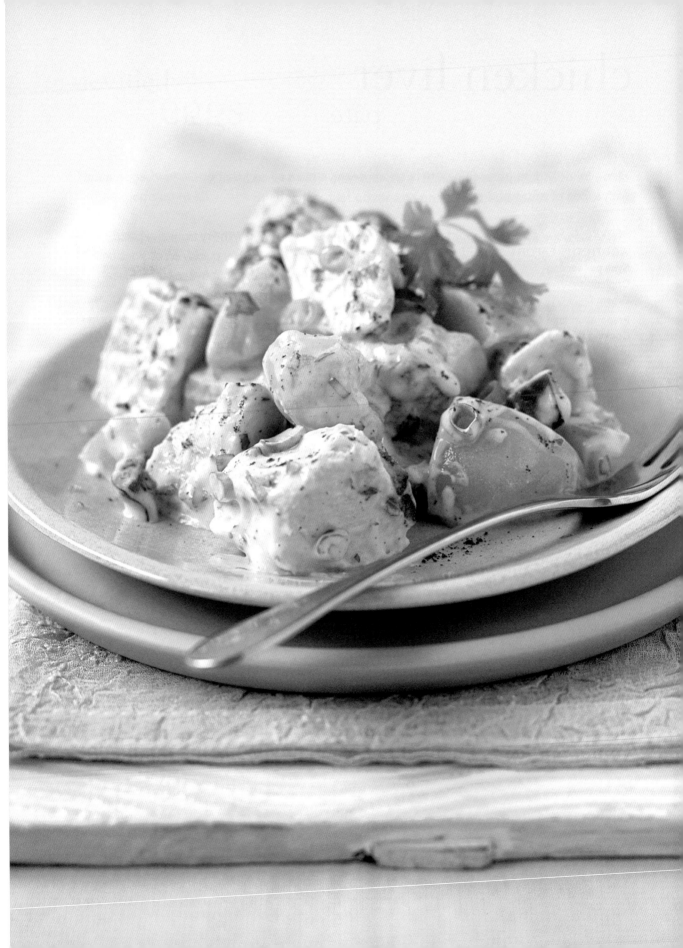

coronation chicken

For a special occasion this salad can be turned into an attractive starter by serving it inside crisp Little Gem lettuce leaves.

SERVES 4

EASY

Syns per serving
Original: 2½
Green: 15

Preparation time 15 minutes

4 large cooked chicken breasts, skinless and cut into bite-sized pieces

1 red pepper, deseeded and cut into 1.5cm/¾in dice

400g/14oz mango, diced

2 tbsp mango chutney

6 tbsp extra light mayonnaise

2 tsp curry powder, plus extra for dusting

200g/7oz very low fat natural yogurt

juice and finely grated zest of 1 lime

salt and freshly ground black pepper

6 spring onions, very finely sliced

8 tbsp roughly chopped coriander

To serve
curry powder, to dust

1. Place the chicken in a shallow bowl with the red pepper and diced mango.

2. In a separate bowl mix together the chutney, mayonnaise, curry powder, yogurt and the lime juice and zest. Season well.

3. Pour the mayonnaise mixture over the chicken and fruit, then stir in the spring onions and coriander. Toss well and serve dusted with a little curry powder.

chicken
caesar salad

Traditional Caesar salad includes anchovies, but here we use chicken, a less salty and lower-fat option, but still full of flavour.

SERVES 4

WORTH THE EFFORT

Syns per serving
Original: 6
Green: 22½

Preparation time 20 minutes
Cooking time 10–12 minutes for the croutons

4 cooked chicken breasts, skinless and cut into bite-sized pieces

2 red apples, cored and cut into bite-sized pieces

4 sticks celery, thinly sliced

1 head of cos or romaine lettuce, washed and roughly torn

6 spring onions, finely sliced

4 tbsp finely chopped chives

4 tbsp light/reduced fat Caesar-style dressing

For the croutons

4 medium slices wholemeal bread, cut into 1.5cm/¾in cubes

4 tsp garlic salt

4 tsp dried parsley

Fry Light

To serve

2 hard-boiled eggs, peeled and finely chopped

8 lean bacon rashers, grilled until crisp

1. Preheat the oven to 200°C/Gas 6. Place the bread for the croutons in a bowl and sprinkle over the garlic salt and parsley. Spray with Fry Light and toss to coat evenly. Place the cubes on a baking sheet in a single layer and bake for 10–12 minutes, or until lightly browned and crisp. Set aside.

2. Place the chicken in a large salad bowl with the apples, celery, lettuce, spring onions and chives. Pour the dressing over the mixture and toss well.

3. Scatter the salad with the chopped eggs, crumble the grilled bacon over, and top with the garlic croutons before serving.

barbecue chicken wings

Marinated ahead of time with flavoursome ingredients, these chicken wings can be cooked quickly and they're finger-lickin' good!

SERVES 4 ✳

EASY

Syns per serving

Original: ½

Green: 19

Preparation time 15 minutes
plus marinating

Cooking time 15–20 minutes

16 large chicken wings, skinless

10 tbsp dark soy sauce

1 tbsp runny honey

2 tbsp garlic salt

2 tsp ground ginger

2 tbsp passata

4 tbsp white wine vinegar

1. Place the chicken wings in a shallow, ceramic bowl.

2. In a separate bowl whisk together the soy sauce, honey, garlic salt, ginger, passata and vinegar. Pour this mixture over the chicken and toss well to coat evenly. Cover and chill for 6–8 hours, or overnight if time permits.

3. Preheat the grill or barbecue until medium hot. Place the chicken on a rack and cook for 15–20 minutes, turning often, until it is cooked through. Serve immediately.

prawn
cocktail

A timeless classic, this colourful and tasty starter will always be very much in demand. It also makes a delicious light lunch.

SERVES 4

EASY

Syns per serving

Original: 1

Green: 9

Preparation time 15 minutes

600g/1lb 6oz cooked, peeled prawns

6 tbsp extra light mayonnaise

2 tbsp passata

a few drops of Tabasco sauce

juice of 1 lemon

100g/3½oz very low fat natural fromage frais

salt and freshly ground black pepper

100g/3½oz iceberg lettuce, very finely shredded

To serve

freshly chopped chives and dill

paprika

1. Place the prawns in a bowl, reserving 4 for decoration. Mix together the mayonnaise, passata, Tabasco, lemon juice and fromage frais in a small bowl and add seasoning. Pour this mixture over the prawns and toss well.

2. Divide the shredded lettuce between 4 bowls or cocktail glasses, then spoon in the prawn mixture. Garnish with the chopped herbs, the reserved prawns and a dusting of paprika, and serve immediately.

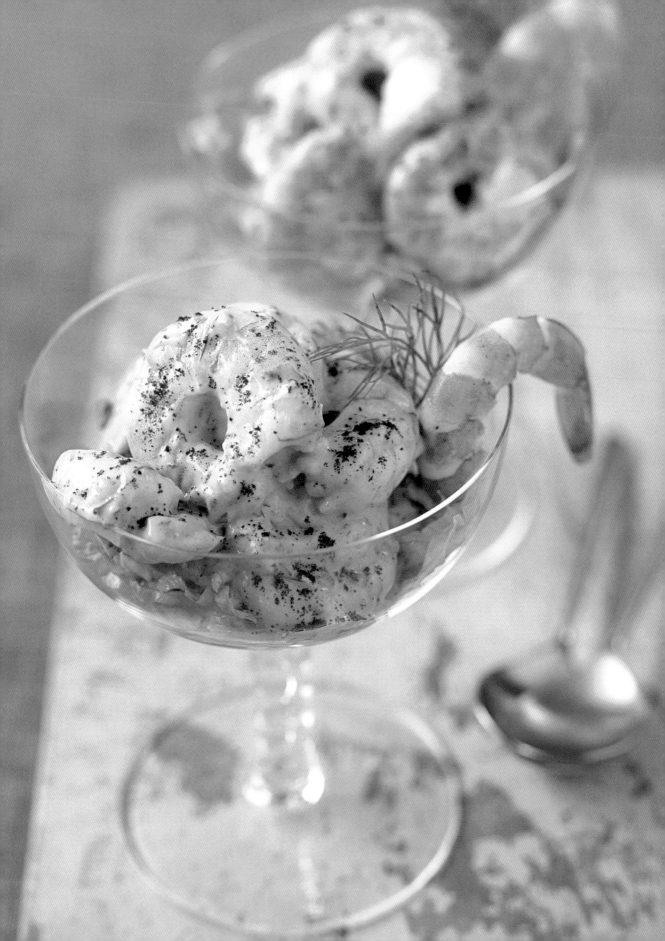

avocado
and prawns

Here's an old favourite that's always popular. For a retro look you could serve this starter in the scooped-out avocado shells.

SERVES 4

EASY

Syns per serving
Original: 8
Green: 9½

Preparation time 15 minutes

2 avocados

150g/5oz good-quality prawns, cooked and peeled

4 tomatoes, skinned, deseeded and diced

For the cocktail sauce

6 tbsp extra light mayonnaise

juice of 1 lemon

2 tbsp passata

1 tsp Worcestershire sauce

a few drops of Tabasco sauce

2 tbsp chopped dill

salt and freshly ground black pepper

1. Whisk all the sauce ingredients together in a small bowl. Season well and set aside.

2. Halve the avocados lengthways and remove the stones. Scoop out the flesh and roughly dice. Season well and mix with 1 or 2 tablespoons of the sauce.

3. Half fill 4 cocktail glasses with the avocado mixture. Mix the prawns and tomatoes together, season to taste, then pile on top of the avocado. Spoon over the cocktail sauce and serve immediately.

moules marinière

Mussels are readily available almost all year round, so make the most of them. This classic French way of cooking them quickly with wine and garlic is simple yet very impressive.

SERVES 4

WORTH THE EFFORT

Syns per serving
Original: 1
Green: 8

Preparation time 15–20 minutes
Cooking time 5–6 minutes

2kg/4lb 8oz fresh, live mussels

6 garlic cloves, peeled and finely chopped

4 shallots, peeled and very finely chopped

1 fresh bay leaf

1 tbsp crushed fennel seeds

100ml/3½fl oz dry white wine

200ml/7fl oz hot stock made with Chicken Bovril

100g/3½oz very low fat natural fromage frais

To serve

4 tbsp finely chopped flat-leaf parsley

salt and freshly ground black pepper

1. Scrub the mussels, discarding any open ones, and remove the 'beards'. Place the mussels, garlic, shallots, bay leaf, fennel seeds, wine and stock in a large saucepan and place over a high heat. Cover tightly and cook for 5–6 minutes, shaking the pan frequently, until all the mussels have opened. Discard the bay leaf and any mussels that remain closed.

2. Drain the mussels, reserving any juices, and divide between 4 warmed bowls. Mix the fromage frais into the reserved juices and spoon over the mussels. Garnish with the chopped parsley, season and serve immediately.

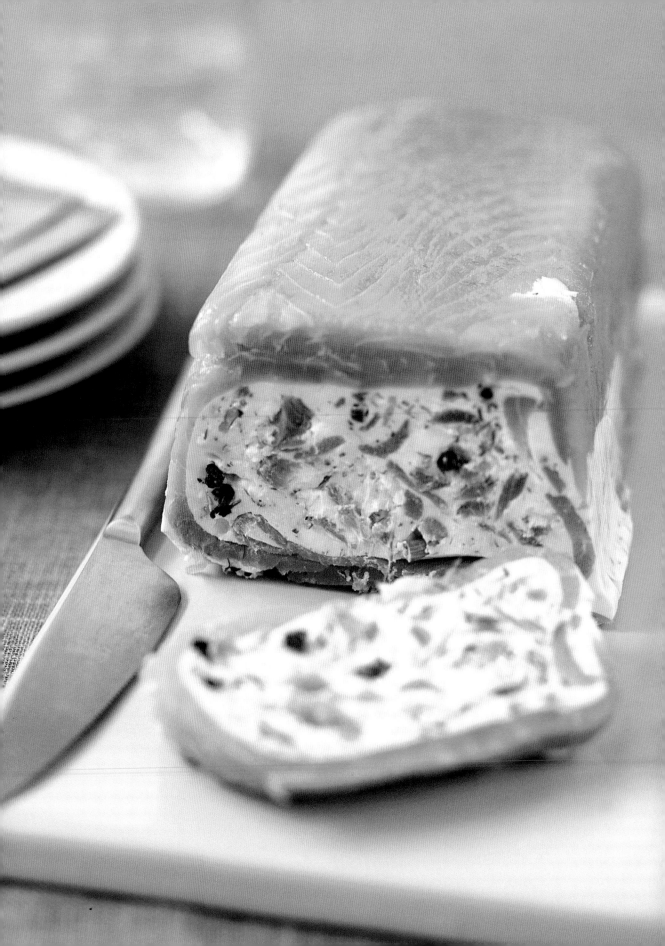

smoked salmon
terrine

This elegant and attractive starter, which is prepared ahead of time, will wow your guests and make for easy entertaining.

SERVES 4

WORTH THE EFFORT

Syns per serving
Original: Free
Green: 9

Preparation time 25 minutes
plus chilling

500g/1lb 2oz smoked salmon slices

15g/½oz powdered gelatine

200ml/7fl oz hot stock made with Chicken Bovril

2 garlic cloves, peeled and crushed

6 tbsp finely chopped dill

200g/7oz quark

2 tbsp pink peppercorns

juice of 1 lemon

salt and freshly ground black pepper

1. Line a small loaf tin with cling film, then line with overlapping slices of half the smoked salmon, making sure that the top ones overhang the sides of the tin.

2. Sprinkle the gelatine over the hot stock and stir to dissolve completely.

3. Roughly chop the remaining salmon and place in a food processor with the garlic, dill, quark, peppercorns and lemon juice. Pour in the gelatine liquid, season well and process until smooth. Spoon this mixture into the lined tin, and enclose with the overhanging salmon slices. Cover and refrigerate overnight or until set.

4. To serve, carefully turn out the terrine, peel away the cling film and cut into thick slices.

salmon
gravadlax

This stunningly coloured salmon is 'cured' for two and a half days in the fridge in a mixture of dill, juniper berries and beetroot. Try to use the freshest wild organic salmon you can get.

SERVES 4

WORTH THE EFFORT

Syns per serving
Original: Free
Green: 20½

Preparation time 20 minutes plus curing

1 thick fresh salmon fillet, about 900g/2lb, skin on
2 medium-sized raw beetroot
100g/3½oz sea salt
6–8 tbsp artificial sweetener
2 tsp freshly ground black pepper
2–3 juniper berries, crushed
150g/5oz fresh dill, chopped

To serve
sprigs of dill

1. Trim the salmon into a neat shape. Feeling with your fingertips and using tweezers, pull out any bones. Place the fillet in a shallow dish, skin-side down.

2. Peel and coarsely grate the beetroot into a bowl (wear rubber gloves to prevent your fingers getting stained). Mix in the salt, sweetener, black pepper, juniper berries and half the dill. Press this mixture evenly all over the salmon, cover with cling film and weigh it down by placing a plate on top (this will help the cure to stick to the flesh). Refrigerate for 24 hours. The cure will cause liquid to seep out of the salmon, but don't drain it away; it will help cure the underside of the fish too.

3. After 24 hours, scrape the beetroot mixture off the salmon, wash the flesh under cold water and pat dry with kitchen paper. Sprinkle with the rest of the dill, wrap firmly in cling film and refrigerate for another 6–8 hours.

4. Using a long, sharp knife, carve the salmon into slices 1cm/½in thick. Arrange on a platter, garnish with sprigs of dill and serve.

smoked mackerel pâté

The rich flavour of smoked mackerel is a perfect foil for the creaminess of this pâté. To ring the changes try using any other smoked fish, such as trout or salmon, instead.

SERVES 4

EASY

Syns per serving
Original: 4
Green: 17½

Preparation time 15 minutes
plus chilling

2 smoked mackerel, skinless
and boneless

125g/4½oz very low fat natural
cottage cheese

150g/5oz quark

juice of ½ a lemon

4 tbsp finely chopped dill

¼ tsp grated nutmeg

salt and freshly ground black
pepper

To serve

cayenne pepper

lemon wedges

1. Flake the mackerel and place in a food processor with the cottage cheese, quark, lemon juice, dill and nutmeg. Season to taste and blend until smooth.

2. Divide the mixture between 4 individual ramekins. Cover with cling film and chill for 2 hours. Just before serving, sprinkle with a little cayenne pepper and garnish with the lemon wedges.

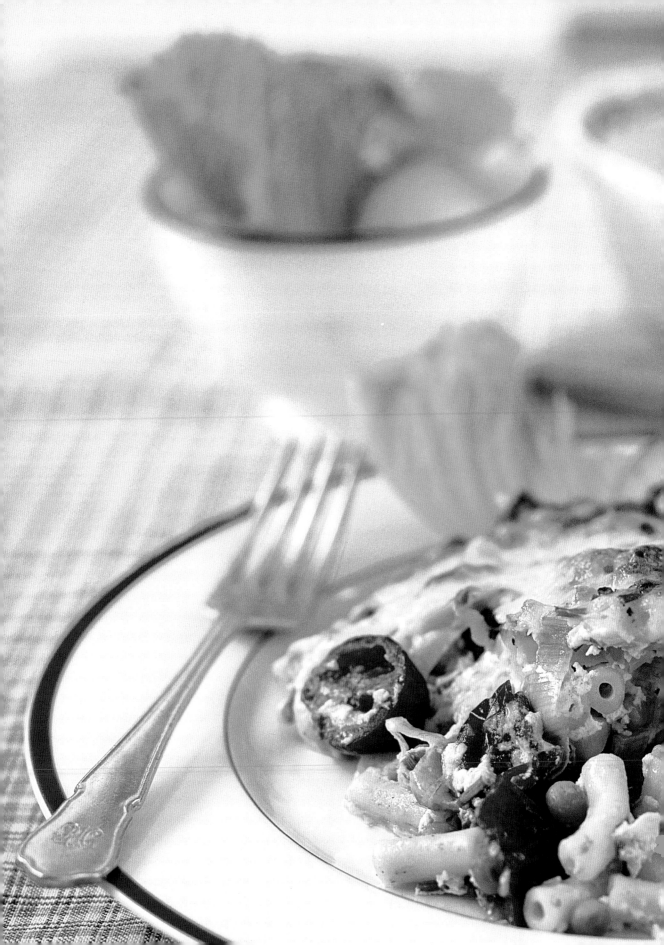

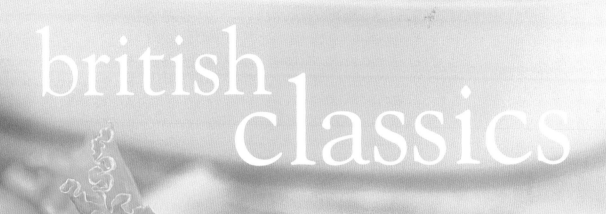

british
classics

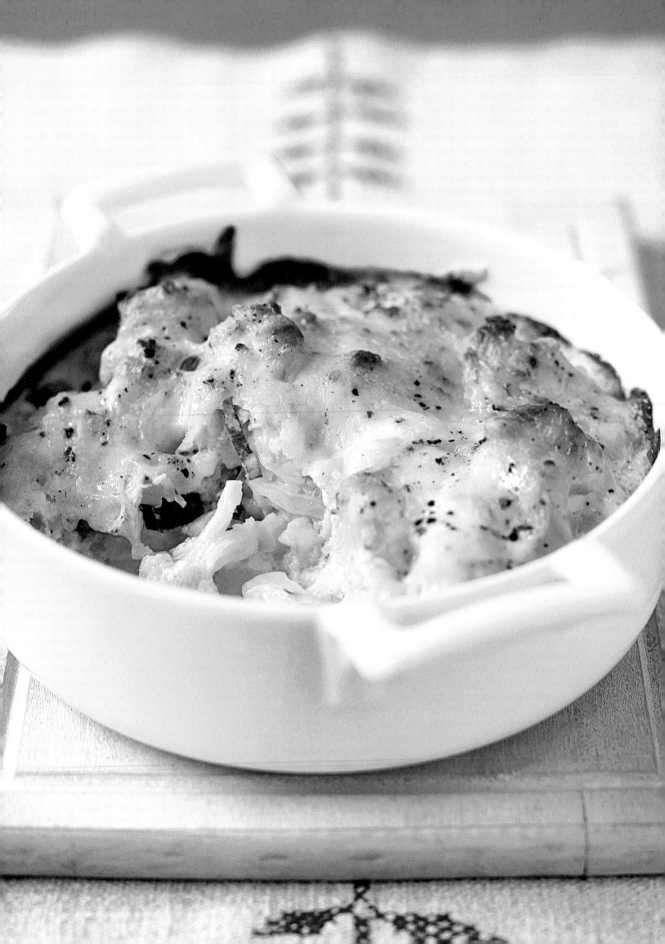

cauliflower cheese

This childhood favourite is best served with a crisp green salad or as an accompaniment to grilled fish or chicken.

SERVES 4 Ⓥ ❋
EASY
Syns per serving
Original: 6
Green: 6

Preparation time 6–8 minutes
Cooking time about 30 minutes, plus standing

6 spring onions, thinly sliced

2 garlic cloves, peeled and chopped

800g/1lb 12oz cauliflower florets, boiled and drained

For the topping

500g/1lb 2oz very low fat natural yogurt

1 tsp Dijon mustard

175g/6oz reduced fat Cheddar cheese, coarsely grated

2 eggs, lightly beaten

salt and freshly ground black pepper

1. Place a large, non-stick frying pan over a high heat. Add the spring onions, garlic and cauliflower and 100ml/3½fl oz of water to the pan and cook for 5–7 minutes, until the water has been absorbed. Mix well, then transfer to a shallow, ovenproof dish.

2. Preheat the oven to 220°C/Gas 7. Put all the topping ingredients in a bowl, season well and mix together. Pour over the cauliflower mixture, then place in the oven and bake for 15–20 minutes, or until lightly golden and bubbling. Remove and allow to stand for 5 minutes before serving.

bangers and mash
with onion gravy

The simplest dishes are often the best, and this classic combination proves the point. Our version of bangers and mash makes a great lunch or dinner.

SERVES 4 Ⓥ ❋
EASY
Syns per serving
Green: 1½
Original: 9½

Preparation time 10–15 minutes
Cooking time about 45 minutes

12 Quorn sausages

For the mash

900g/2lb Desirée potatoes, peeled and chopped

1 tsp English mustard powder

200g/7oz very low fat natural fromage frais

salt and freshly ground black pepper

For the gravy

Fry Light

6 onions, peeled, halved and very finely sliced

500ml/18fl oz water or stock made with Vecon

1 tbsp onion gravy granules

1 tsp dried mixed herbs

1. Start by making the gravy. Spray a large, non-stick frying pan with Fry Light and place it over a medium heat. Add the onions and stir-fry for 2–3 minutes. Reduce the heat to low and cook gently, stirring occasionally, for 15–20 minutes, or until the onions are lightly coloured and soft.

2. Pour in the water or stock, add the gravy granules and dried herbs and bring to the boil. Lower the heat and cook gently for 15–20 minutes, or until the gravy has thickened. Remove from the heat and keep warm.

3. While the gravy is cooking, make the mash. Put the potatoes in a large saucepan of lightly salted boiling water and cook for 15–20 minutes, or until very tender. Drain and return to the pan. Mix together the mustard powder and fromage frais, stir into the potatoes, then mash until well blended and smooth. Season well and keep warm.

4. About 5 minutes before the potatoes are tender, spray a large, non-stick frying pan with Fry Light and place over a medium heat. Fry the sausages for 8–10 minutes, or until cooked through and browned. Serve with the mash and gravy.

cottage pie

This comforting family bake is perfect for a rainy day. As it freezes well, it can be made in advance and heated through whenever you need it.

SERVES 4 ⓥ ❋

EASY

Syns per serving

Green: Free

Original: 8½

Preparation time 20 minutes

Cooking time 50 minutes

900g/2lb potatoes, peeled and chopped

6 tbsp very low fat natural yogurt

4 tbsp chopped parsley

salt and freshly ground black pepper

Fry Light

1 red onion, peeled and finely chopped

2 garlic cloves, peeled and crushed

2 sticks celery, finely chopped

2 carrots, peeled and finely chopped

350g/12oz Quorn mince

1 x 400g can chopped tomatoes

1 tbsp Vecon

1 tsp artificial sweetener

2 tsp dried oregano

1 egg, lightly beaten

1. Put the potatoes in a pan of lightly salted boiling water and cook for about 15–20 minutes, or until tender. Drain, return to the pan and mash until smooth. Stir in the yogurt and parsley, season well and set aside.

2. While the potatoes are cooking, spray a large frying pan with Fry Light and place over a high heat. Add the onion, garlic, celery and carrots and stir-fry for 4–5 minutes. Add the Quorn mince and stir-fry for 4–5 minutes. Add the tomatoes, Vecon, sweetener and oregano and stir well. Bring to the boil and remove from the heat.

3. Preheat the oven to 200°C/Gas 6. Transfer the vegetable mixture to a medium-sized pie dish and top with the potato mixture. Ruffle the surface with a fork, brush with the beaten egg and bake for 25–30 minutes, until lightly golden and bubbling. Serve immediately with vegetables of your choice.

luxury macaroni cheese

So delicious, it's hard to believe that this is a low-fat dish. Leeks, cherry tomatoes and chives add wonderful extra flavour to this favourite, family-style bake.

SERVES 4 Ⓥ ❆
EASY
Syns per serving
Green: 6
Original: 11½

Preparation time 15 minutes
Cooking time about 30 minutes
plus standing

2 leeks, thinly sliced

2 garlic cloves, peeled and chopped

300g/11oz cherry tomatoes, halved

200g/7oz frozen peas

2 tbsp finely chopped chives

100ml/3½fl oz water

400g/14oz cooked macaroni or other short-shape pasta

For the topping

500g/1lb 2oz very low fat natural yogurt

1 tsp Dijon mustard

175g/6oz reduced fat Cheddar cheese, coarsely grated

2 eggs, lightly beaten

4 tbsp very finely chopped parsley

salt and freshly ground black pepper

1. Place a large, non-stick frying pan over a high heat. Add the leeks, garlic, tomatoes, peas, chives and water, stir together and cook for 6–8 minutes, until the water has been absorbed.

2. Stir the cooked pasta into the tomato mixture, then transfer to a shallow, ovenproof dish.

3. Preheat the oven to 220°C/Gas 7. Mix all the topping ingredients in a bowl, season well and pour over the pasta mixture. Place in the oven and cook for 15–20 minutes, or until lightly golden and bubbling. Allow to stand for 5 minutes before serving. Accompany with a crisp green salad.

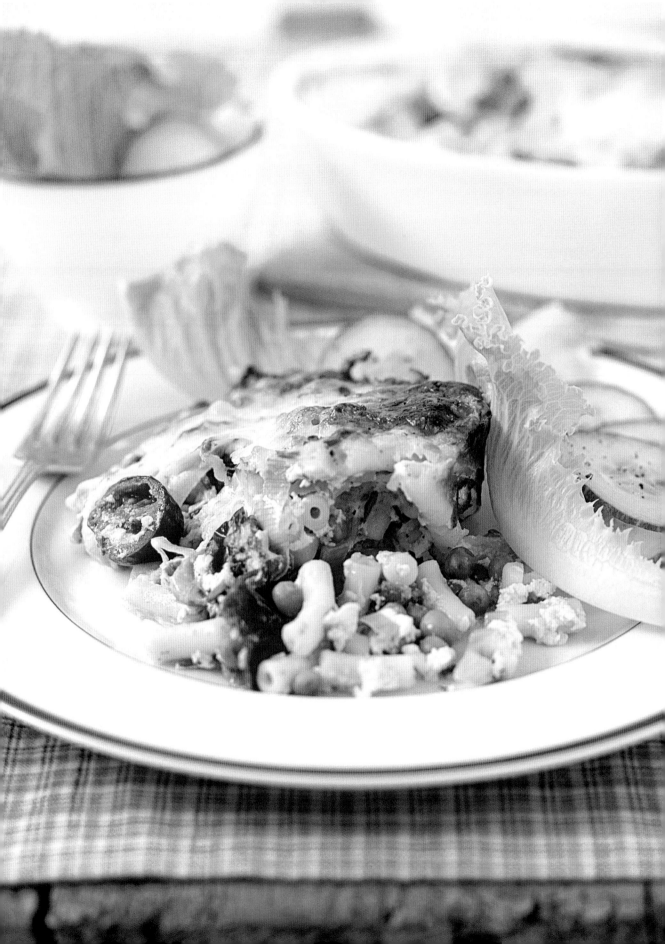

classic
new potato salad

This versatile salad is perfect for lazy summer entertaining and, as it travels well, it makes terrific picnic fare.

SERVES 4 ⓥ

EASY

Syns per serving
Green: 2
Original: 9½

Preparation time 10–15 minutes
Cooking time 15–20 minutes

800g/1lb 12oz new potatoes

2 red apples, cored and cut into bite-sized pieces

1 small red onion, peeled and finely chopped

4 spring onions, finely sliced

8 tbsp finely chopped dill

4 tbsp finely snipped chives

4–5 tbsp finely chopped gherkins

For the dressing

8 tbsp extra light mayonnaise

3 tbsp wine vinegar

1 tsp runny honey

1 tbsp Dijon or wholegrain mustard

salt and freshly ground black pepper

1. Cut the potatoes into halves, or bite-sized pieces if large, and boil in lightly salted water until tender. Drain and place in a large mixing bowl with the apples, red onion, spring onions, dill, chives and gherkins.

2. Combine all the dressing ingredients, add seasoning and pour over the potato mixture. Stir well and serve warm or at room temperature.

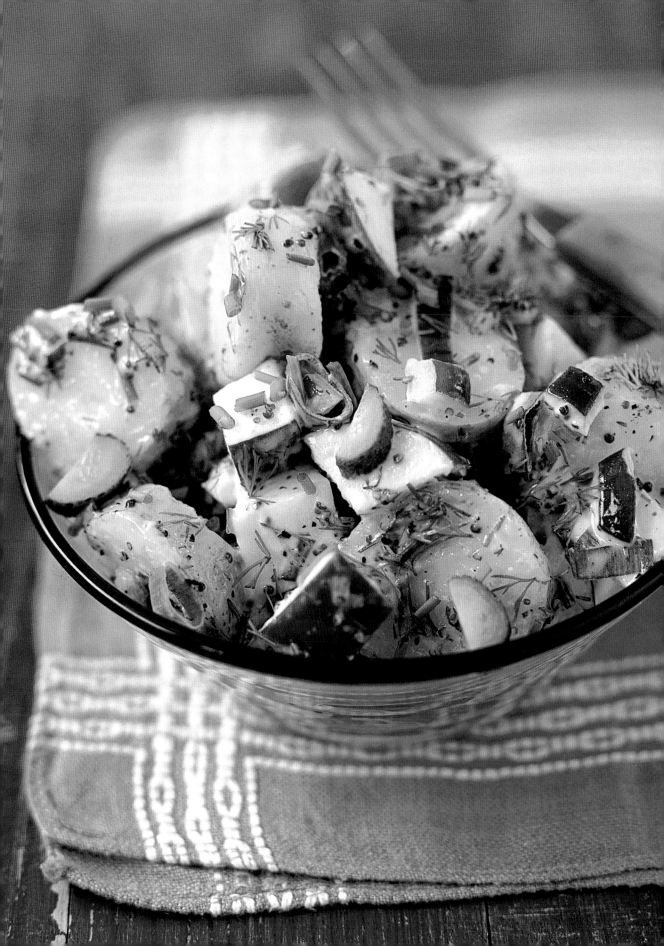

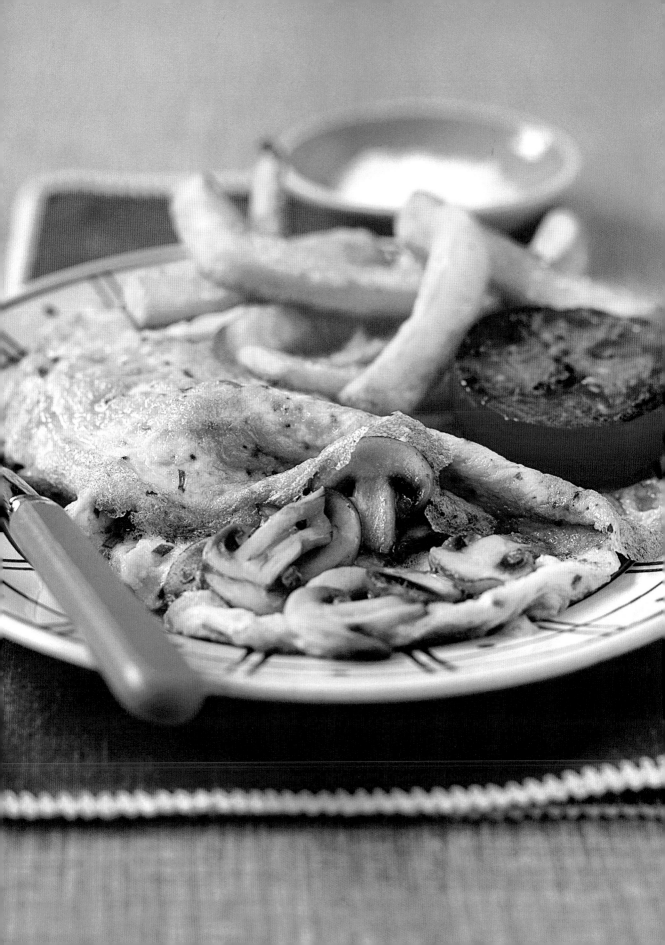

slimming world chips and best ever mushroom omelette

You can experiment with all kinds of fillings for an omelette and also vary the chopped herbs used to season it. On an Original day add cooked lean bacon to the mushroom mixture to give extra flavour.

CHIPS SERVE 4 ⓥ
OMELETTE SERVES 1 ⓥ
EASY

Syns per serving

Chips

Green: Free

Original: 7½

Omelette

Green: Free

Original: Free

Preparation time about 20 minutes

Cooking time about 35 minutes

800g/1lb 12oz large potatoes, peeled

Fry Light

sea salt

For the omelette

2 large eggs

2 tbsp finely chopped chives

2 tbsp finely chopped parsley

1 tsp cold water

salt and freshly ground black pepper

200g/7oz sliced, cooked mushrooms

To serve

grilled tomatoes

1. Preheat the oven to 190°C/Gas 5. Cut the potatoes into chunky, even-sized chips and place in a large pan of lightly salted boiling water. Boil for 6–7 minutes, then drain thoroughly. Return to the pan, replace the lid and shake to roughen the edges of the chips (this helps them to crisp up during baking).

2. Line a baking sheet with non-stick baking parchment and spread out the chips. Spray with Fry Light and sprinkle with sea salt. Place in the oven and bake for 15–20 minutes, or until the chips are crisp and golden.

3. About 5 minutes before the chips are ready, gently beat the eggs together with the herbs and water. Season well.

4. Spray a medium, non-stick frying pan with a thin coating of Fry Light and place over a high heat. When hot, pour in the egg mixture and cook for 1–2 minutes. As the egg begins to set around the edges, add the cooked mushrooms and use a spatula to push the egg towards the centre. When the entire egg mixture is set, cook for another minute, then loosen the edges with a spatula and fold the omelette in half. Serve with the chips and grilled tomatoes.

pan haggerty

Originally from Northumberland, this potato and onion 'cake' is a nutritious and economical supper dish. We include cabbage in our version, which makes it a complete meal in a pan.

SERVES 4 Ⓥ ❈
EASY
Syns per serving
Green: Free
Original: 9½

Preparation time 20 minutes
Cooking time about 45 minutes

1kg/2lb 4oz Desirée potatoes, peeled and roughly chopped

400g/14oz cabbage, finely shredded

2 large eggs, lightly beaten

2 garlic cloves, peeled and crushed

2 onions, peeled, halved and finely sliced

salt and freshly ground black pepper

Fry Light

1. Cook the potatoes in a large saucepan of lightly salted boiling water until just tender. Drain thoroughly, return to the saucepan and add the cabbage. Allow the mixture to cool, then add the eggs, garlic and onions. Season well and mix thoroughly.

2. When ready to cook, preheat the oven to 180°C/Gas 4. Spray a large, ovenproof frying pan with Fry Light. Spoon the potato mixture into the pan, pressing down to form a smooth 'cake'. Bake in the oven for 25–30 minutes, or until lightly golden. Serve immediately.

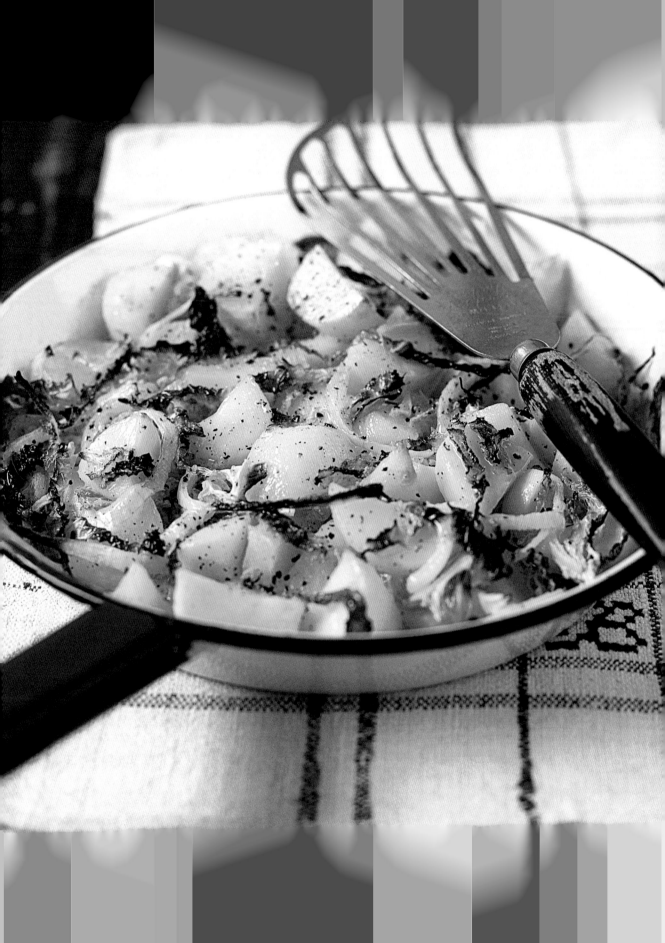

bubble
and squeak

Leftover potato and cabbage are the traditional basis of this British favourite. For a change, the mixture can be shaped into little cakes and baked to serve as snacks.

SERVES 4 Ⓥ ❄
EASY
Syns per serving
Green: Free
Original: 6

Preparation time 10 minutes
Cooking time about 25 minutes

500g/1lb 2oz Savoy cabbage, finely shredded

600g/1lb 6oz potatoes, peeled and finely chopped

Fry Light

4 spring onions, finely sliced

1 tsp wholegrain mustard

150g/5oz very low fat natural fromage frais

salt and freshly ground black pepper

To serve

freshly grated nutmeg

1. Cook the cabbage and potatoes in a large saucepan of lightly salted boiling water for 12–15 minutes, or until the potatoes are tender. Drain thoroughly.

2. Spray a large, non-stick wok or frying pan with Fry Light and place over a high heat. Add the spring onions and the potato mixture and stir-fry for 6–8 minutes. Stir in the mustard and fromage frais. Remove from the heat, season and serve sprinkled with the nutmeg.

luxury fish pie

Ultimate comfort food, this fish pie has a carrot and swede mash topping, making it Free on an Original day.

SERVES 4 ❋

WORTH THE EFFORT

Syns per serving
Original: Free
Green: 6½

Preparation time 30 minutes
Cooking time under 1 hour

300g/11oz very low fat natural yogurt

150g/5oz quark

4 tbsp finely chopped dill

2 tbsp chopped parsley

6 hard-boiled eggs, peeled and cut in half

200g/7oz cod fillets, cooked, skinned and cut into large bite-sized

pieces

200g/7oz smoked haddock fillets, cooked, skinned and flaked

200g/7oz cooked peeled prawns

juice of ½ lemon

For the topping

400g/14oz carrots, peeled and roughly chopped

300g/11oz swede, peeled and roughly chopped

1 large egg, beaten

4 tbsp very low fat natural yogurt

salt and freshly ground black pepper

1. Start by making the topping. Put the carrots and swede in a large pan of lightly salted boiling water and cook for 25–30 minutes, until tender. Drain, return to the pan and mash. Allow to cool. Stir in the beaten egg and yogurt, season and set aside.

2. Preheat the oven to 200°C/Gas 6. Mix together the yogurt, quark, dill and parsley. Season well and set aside.

3. Place the hard-boiled eggs, cod, haddock, prawns and lemon juice in a large mixing bowl. Pour over the quark mixture, season and mix well. Transfer this mixture to a deep, ovenproof dish. Spoon the topping evenly over the surface, then ruffle with a fork. Place in the oven and bake for 20–25 minutes, until the topping is lightly browned. Serve immediately with steamed green vegetables.

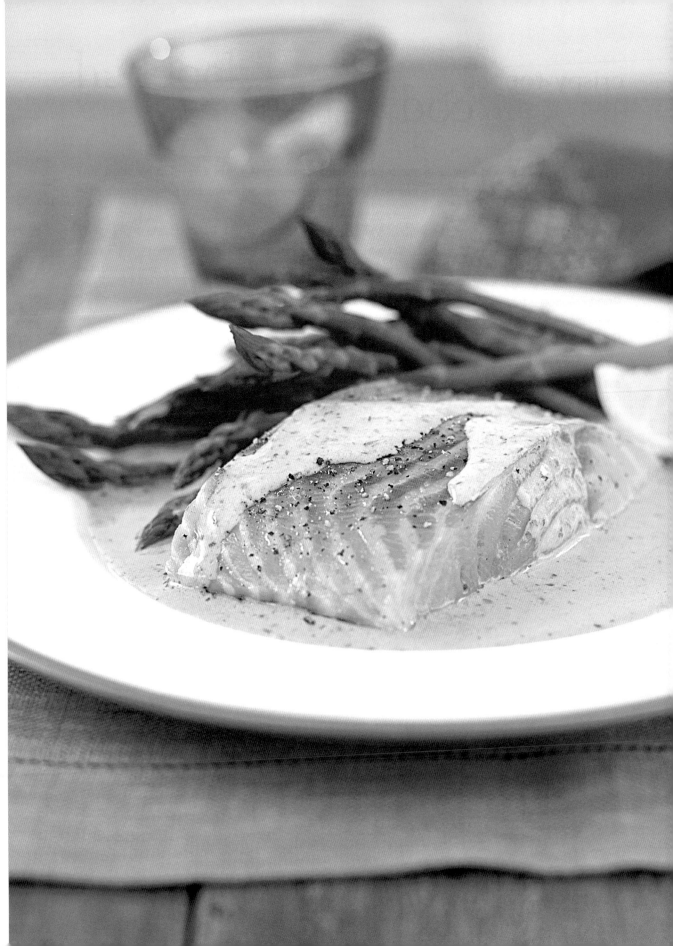

salmon
with parsley sauce

The distinctive taste of fresh salmon fillets lends itself very well to a savoury, herb-flavoured sauce.

SERVES 4

EXTRA EASY

Syns per serving
Original: Free
Green: 15½

Preparation time 20 minutes
Cooking time about 10 minutes

4 large salmon fillets, skinless

For the parsley sauce

100g/3½oz parsley, roughly chopped

200g/7oz very low fat natural fromage frais

100g/3½oz quark

100ml/3½fl oz stock made with Chicken Bovril

4 tbsp capers, rinsed and chopped

salt and freshly ground black pepper

1. Start by making the sauce. Place the parsley, fromage frais, quark, stock and capers in a food processor and blend until smooth. Season well, transfer to a bowl and set aside until ready to serve.

2. Preheat the grill until hot. Place the salmon fillets on a rack in a single layer and season well. Grill for 8–10 minutes, or until the fish has cooked through.

3. Place each fillet on a warmed plate, spoon over the sauce and serve with asparagus, if wished.

baked
trout

Really fresh fish is one of life's great pleasures. Here the aromatic flavours of garlic, lemon and parsley complement the delicate flavour of trout.

SERVES 4

EXTRA EASY

Syns per serving
Original: Free
Green: 12½

Preparation time 5 minutes
Cooking time 20 minutes

4 rainbow trout, gutted and cleaned

salt and freshly ground black pepper

2 garlic cloves, peeled and finely chopped

juice and finely grated zest of 2 lemons

4 tbsp finely chopped parsley

Fry Light

1. Preheat the oven to 200°C/Gas 6. Season the fish well inside and out and place in a non-stick roasting tin. Sprinkle over the garlic, lemon juice, zest and half the parsley. Spray with Fry Light and bake in the oven for 20 minutes, or until the fish is cooked through.

2. Remove from the oven and sprinkle over the remaining parsley. Serve immediately with grilled vine tomatoes.

grilled dover sole
with horseradish cream

This might sound like an unusual combination, but the hot flavour of creamy horseradish goes extremely well with simply grilled fish.

SERVES 4

EXTRA EASY

Syns per serving
Original: ½
Green: 13

Preparation time 5 minutes
Cooking time about 10 minutes

8 Dover sole fillets, skinless
Fry Light
salt and freshly ground black pepper

For the horseradish cream
1 tbsp creamed horseradish
150g/5oz quark
100g/3½oz very low fat natural fromage frais

1. Preheat the grill until very hot. Place the fish fillets on a rack in a single layer, spray with Fry Light and season well. Grill for 8–10 minutes, or until the fish is cooked through.

2. Meanwhile, make the horseradish cream by mixing all the ingredients in a bowl until smooth. Season well and serve alongside the grilled fish.

the ultimate christmas dinner

lemon and herb roast turkey

The perfect centrepiece for any Christmas meal, this moist and juicy turkey receives a boost of flavour from herbs, garlic, lemon and mustard.

SERVES 8

WORTH THE EFFORT

Syns per serving
Original: ½
Green: 37½

Preparation time 30 minutes
Cooking time under 3 hours, plus resting

1 x 5.5kg/12lb 6oz oven-ready turkey
4 tbsp dried mixed herbs
juice of 2 lemons
1 tbsp Dijon mustard
Fry Light
2 lemons, halved
1 onion, halved
2 heads of garlic, unpeeled and halved across the centre
a small bunch of thyme sprigs

For the gravy
1 tbsp turkey gravy granules
salt and freshly ground black pepper

1. Preheat the oven to 180°C/Gas 4. Place the turkey in a large, non-stick roasting tin. Put the herbs, lemon juice and mustard in a small bowl, mix together, then spread over the turkey. Spray Fry Light all over the bird. Fill the body cavity with the lemon halves, onion, garlic and thyme and tie the legs together with string to give a neat shape. Cover loosely with foil and roast in the oven for the appropriate time (see box below). Baste the bird with the pan juices several times during cooking. For the last 30 minutes remove the foil and raise the temperature to 200°C/Gas 6 so that the skin will brown and crisp up.

2. Remove the turkey from the oven, cover with a tent of foil and leave in a warm place to rest (for up to 2 hours) while you cook the rest of the accompaniments.

3. Remove any fat from the roasting liquid, then pour the juices into a saucepan and bring to the boil. Add the gravy granules to thicken the liquid, then season and keep warm.

4. Remove the skin before serving the turkey on a platter, surrounded by Pigs in Blankets, Herbed Stuffing Balls, Brussels Sprouts with Chestnuts, and Glazed Carrots (see pages 78–9).

> **turkey roasting time**
> Allow 45 minutes per 1kg/2lb 4oz, plus 20 minutes.

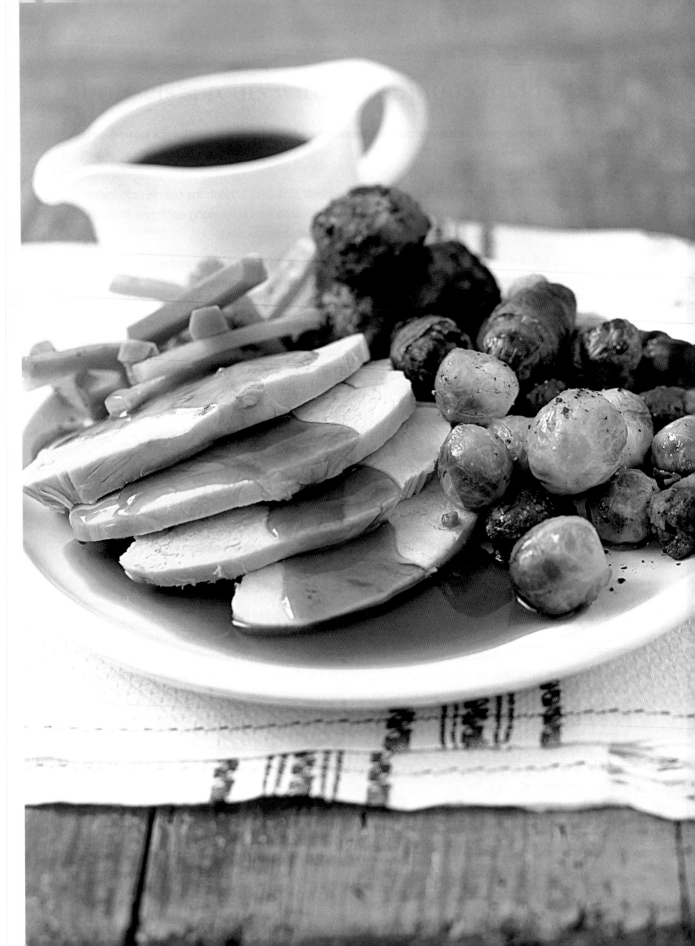

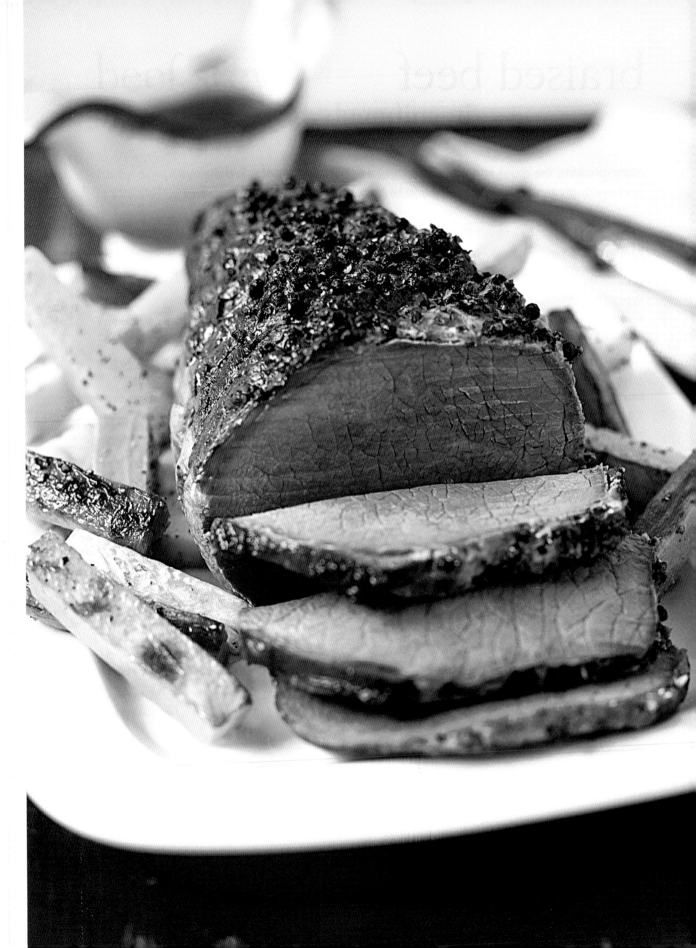

roast rib of beef

with roasted roots and gravy

Here we have the ultimate Sunday lunch, and roasting the vegetables means it's easy to have everything ready at the same time.

SERVES 4

WORTH THE EFFORT

Syns per serving
Original: 1
Green: 20

Preparation time 30 minutes
Cooking time about 1–1½ hours, plus resting

1 x 1.2kg/2lb 10oz rib of beef joint, boneless and all visible fat removed

1 tbsp mustard powder

2 tbsp passata

3 tbsp mixed peppercorns, crushed

400g/14oz swede, peeled and cut into thick pieces

500g/1lb 2oz celeriac, peeled and cut into thick pieces

3 large carrots, peeled and cut into thick batons

For the gravy

400ml/14fl oz stock made with Beef Bovril

1 tbsp cornflour, mixed with cold water to form a paste

1. Preheat the oven to 220°C/Gas 7. Place the beef in a large, non-stick roasting tin. Mix the mustard with the passata until smooth and spread over the beef. Press the crushed peppercorns over this, coating evenly. Place the beef in the oven and roast for 20 minutes, then reduce the heat to 190°C/Gas 5 and roast for a further 30 minutes for rare, 45 minutes for medium rare or 1 hour for well done.

2. Meanwhile, put the vegetables in a large saucepan of lightly salted boiling water and cook for 10 minutes. Drain and add to the roasting tin 20 minutes before the end of the cooking time.

3. To make the gravy, bring the stock to the boil in a small saucepan and add the cornflour paste. Cook for 3–4 minutes, whisking constantly, until thickened. Remove from the heat and keep warm.

4. When the beef is cooked to your liking, remove from the oven, cover and allow to rest for 10–15 minutes before carving. Serve with the roasted vegetables and gravy.

gammon
with egg and pineapple

Mustard powder gives an extra depth of flavour to the gammon steaks and balances out the sweetness of the pineapple.

SERVES 4

WORTH THE EFFORT

Syns per serving
Original: Free
Green: 23½

Preparation time 5 minutes
Cooking time about 25 minutes

8 x 175g/6oz lean gammon steaks
freshly ground black pepper
1 tbsp mustard powder
Fry Light
4 large eggs
8 fresh pineapple rings

To serve
steamed cabbage

1. Preheat a grill until medium hot. Season the gammon steaks with black pepper and the mustard powder. Grill for 4–5 minutes on each side, or until cooked through. Transfer to a plate and keep warm.

2. While the gammon is cooking, spray a large, non-stick frying pan with Fry Light and fry the eggs until done to your liking.

4. To serve, place 2 gammon steaks on a warm plate and top with a couple of pineapple rings and a fried egg. Serve with steamed shredded cabbage.

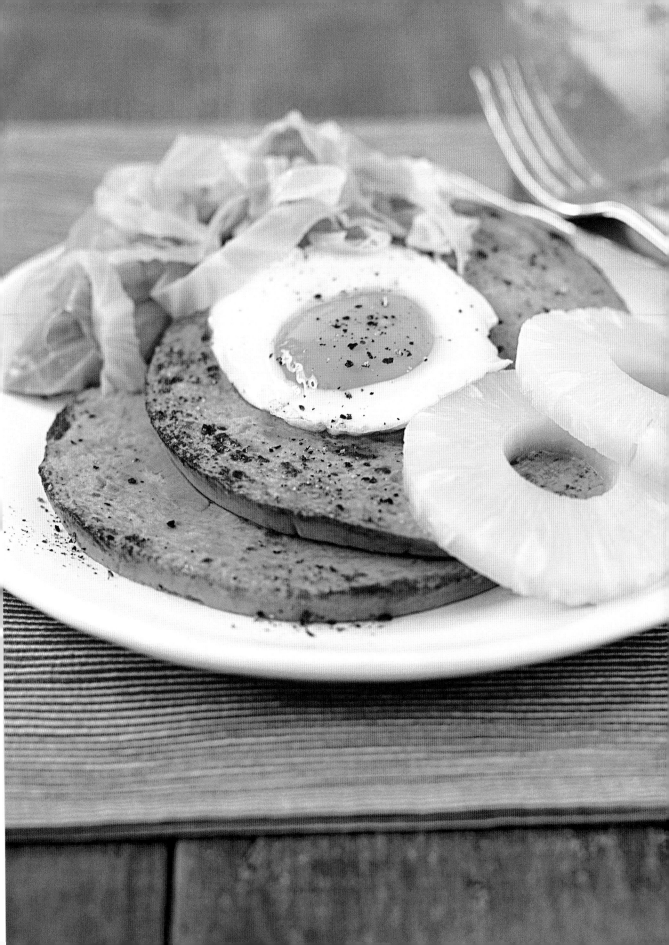

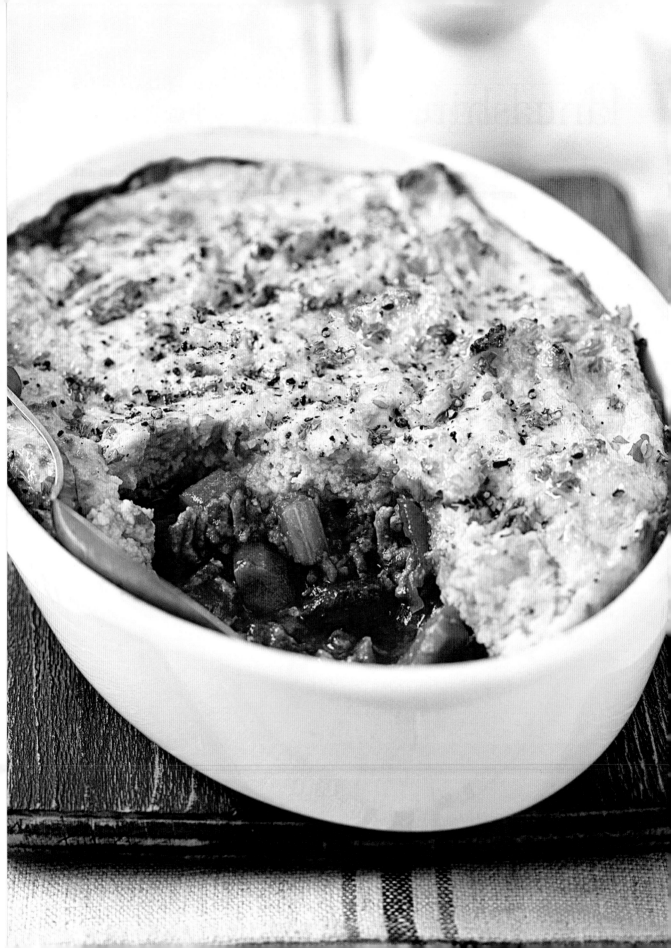

shepherd's pie

If you wish, this recipe can be made into individual pies. Just divide the minced mixture between four individual pie dishes, spoon over the topping and bake for 10–15 minutes.

SERVES 4 ✳
EASY

Syns per serving
Original: Free
Green: 6½

Preparation time 15 minutes
Cooking time 35 minutes

Fry Light

1 red onion, peeled and finely chopped

2 garlic cloves, peeled and crushed

2 sticks celery, finely chopped

2 carrots, peeled and finely chopped

350g/12oz extra-lean lamb mince

1 x 400g can chopped tomatoes

2 tbsp Chicken Bovril

1 tsp artificial sweetener

2 tsp dried oregano

1 egg, beaten

For the topping

500g/18oz swede, peeled and chopped

400g/14oz carrots, peeled and chopped

6 tbsp very low fat natural yogurt

2 egg yolks

4 tbsp chopped parsley

salt and freshly ground black pepper

1. Start by making the topping. Put the swede and carrots in a saucepan of lightly salted boiling water and cook for about 5 minutes, or until tender. Drain, return to the pan and mash until smooth. Stir in the yogurt, egg yolks and parsley, season well and set aside.

2. Meanwhile, spray a large frying pan with Fry Light and place over a high heat. Add the onion, garlic, celery, carrots and lamb mince and stir-fry for 4–5 minutes. Add the tomatoes, Bovril, sweetener and oregano and mix well. Bring to the boil and remove from the heat.

3. Preheat the oven to 200°C/Gas 6. Transfer the mince mixture to a medium pie dish and top with the swede mash, swirling with a fork to ruffle the surface. Brush the beaten egg over the top and bake for 15–20 minutes, until lightly golden and bubbling. Serve immediately.

irish stew

While not strictly British, this dish has become very popular throughout Britain. Garlic, celery, onion and carrots add terrific flavour to this rich and substantial stew.

SERVES 4 ❋
EASY
Syns per serving
Original: 1
Green: 16

Preparation time 20 minutes
Cooking time under 3 hours

800g/1lb 12oz lean neck fillet of lamb, cut into large cubes

3 medium onions, peeled and thickly sliced

2 garlic cloves, peeled and crushed

300g/11oz turnip, peeled and roughly chopped

4 carrots, peeled and roughly chopped

4 sticks celery, roughly chopped

900ml/32fl oz stock made with Chicken Bovril

1 tbsp Chicken Bovril

1 tbsp chicken gravy granules

salt and freshly ground black pepper

To serve

mashed celeriac or swede (optional)

1. Place the lamb, onions, garlic, turnip, carrots and celery in a heavy-based casserole dish. Add the stock, Bovril and gravy granules and bring to the boil. Reduce the heat, season well and mix thoroughly.

2. Cover tightly and cook on a very low heat for 2–2½ hours, or until the lamb is extremely tender. Serve with mashed celeriac or swede, if wished.

one-pot lamb shanks

This hearty and delicious dish is perfect for easy entertaining as it is all cooked in one pot.

SERVES 4 ✽

EASY

Syns per serving

Original: Free

Green: 30½

Preparation time 20 minutes

Cooking time under 3 hours, plus standing

Fry Light

4 lamb shanks, trimmed of all visible fat

1 onion, peeled and finely chopped

2 carrots, peeled and finely chopped

2 sticks celery, finely chopped

4 garlic cloves, peeled and finely chopped

1 x 400g can chopped tomatoes

200ml/7fl oz stock made with Chicken Bovril

1 tsp artificial sweetener (optional)

1 bay leaf

salt and freshly ground black pepper

To serve

finely chopped parsley

finely grated lemon zest

1. Spray a heavy, non-stick casserole with Fry Light and place over a high heat. Add the lamb and lightly brown on all sides. Remove the shanks with a slotted spoon and set aside.

2. Lower the heat to medium and add the onion, carrots, celery and garlic to the casserole. Stir-fry for 10 minutes, then add the tomatoes, stock, sweetener (if using) and bay leaf. Season well. Return the shanks to the casserole, stir and cover tightly. Reduce the heat to very low and cook for 2½ hours, stirring occasionally, until the meat is meltingly tender. Discard the bay leaf and allow to stand for 10 minutes.

3. Spoon the casserole into warmed shallow bowls. Garnish with parsley and lemon zest just before serving.

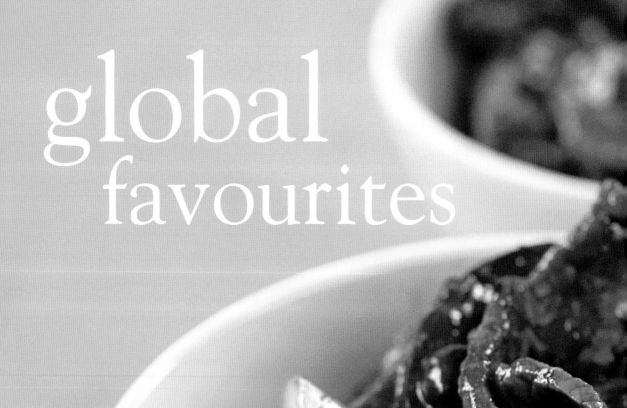

global
favourites

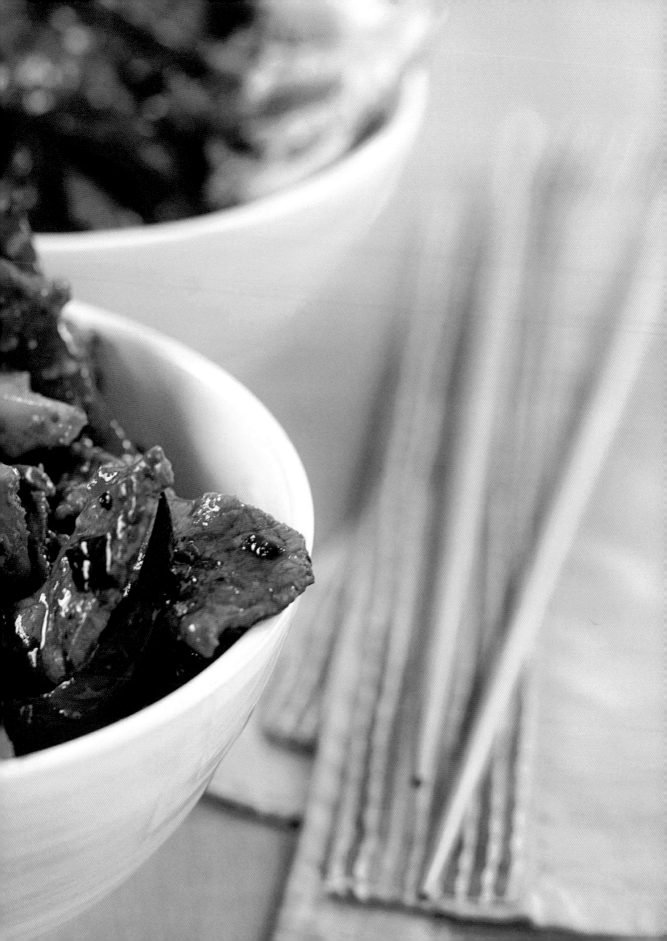

spaghetti bolognese

Bologna is reputed to have the finest cuisine in Italy, and bolognese sauce certainly proves the point. Apart from being absolutely delicious, this version made with Quorn is Free on Slimming World's Green choice, so it's very versatile: serve it on pasta, over rice or spooned into jacket potatoes. It's always a winner!

SERVES 4 Ⓥ ❄ (sauce only)

EASY

Syns per serving
Green: Free
Original: 14½

Preparation time 5 minutes
Cooking time about 35 minutes

Fry Light

1 onion, peeled and finely chopped

3 garlic cloves, peeled and finely chopped

1 tsp cayenne pepper

1 tsp ground cinnamon

500g/1lb 2oz Quorn mince

1 x 400g can chopped tomatoes

4 tbsp finely chopped basil

1 tsp artificial sweetener

salt and freshly ground black pepper

350g/12oz dried spaghetti

To serve

basil leaves

1. Spray a large, non-stick frying pan with Fry Light and place over a medium heat. Add the onion, garlic and cayenne pepper and stir-fry for 2–3 minutes.

2. Add the cinnamon and Quorn to the pan and stir-fry for 3–4 minutes. Add the tomatoes, chopped basil and sweetener and bring to the boil. Season well, cover tightly and cook over a low heat for 20–25 minutes.

3. Meanwhile, cook the spaghetti according to the instructions on the packet. Drain and divide between 4 warmed plates. Spoon the sauce over the top, garnish with basil leaves and serve immediately.

tagliatelle carbonara

Here we have ham, garlic, quark and eggs stirred through hot pasta, creating a creamy and delicious lunch or supper dish. What could be easier?

SERVES 4

EASY

Syns per serving
Green: 5½
Original: 17

Preparation time 5 minutes
Cooking time under 15 minutes

400g/14oz dried tagliatelle
2 eggs
2 egg yolks
50g/2oz quark
salt and freshly ground black pepper
Fry Light
2 garlic cloves, peeled
350g/12oz lean ham, finely diced

To serve

freshly grated Parmesan cheese (optional)

1. Cook the pasta in a large saucepan of lightly salted boiling water until al dente (tender but still retaining a bite). Meanwhile, mix the eggs and egg yolks together, then whisk in the quark until the mixture is smooth. Season and set aside.

2. Spray a large, non-stick frying pan with Fry Light and place over a medium heat. Bruise the garlic with the back of a knife and add to the pan with the ham. Cook over a medium heat for 1–2 minutes.

3. Drain the tagliatelle, add to the frying pan and mix well. Remove the pan from the heat, pour in the egg mixture and toss until the pasta is well coated. Sprinkle over some grated Parmesan (1½ Syns per 1 tbsp), if wished, and serve immediately.

penne arrabbiata

Here is an example of southern Italian cooking, which often incorporates chillies. The word *arrabbiata* means 'angry', and this dish is so called because of its spicy sauce.

SERVES 4 Ⓥ ❋ (sauce only)

EASY

Syns per serving
Green: ½
Original: 17½

Preparation time 10 minutes
Cooking time under 15 minutes

6 spring onions, sliced

14 pitted black olives, sliced

2–3 garlic cloves, peeled and crushed

1 red chilli, deseeded and finely chopped

1 tsp crushed dried red chillies

2 tsp dried oregano

1 x 400g can chopped tomatoes

100ml/3½fl oz water or stock made with Vecon

salt and freshly ground black pepper

400g/14oz dried penne pasta

6 tbsp finely chopped fresh basil

To serve

freshly grated Parmesan cheese (optional)

a few fresh basil leaves

1. Place the spring onions, olives, garlic, chillies, oregano, tomatoes and water or stock in a saucepan and bring to the boil. Lower the heat, season well and cook gently for about 10–12 minutes.

2. While the sauce is simmering, cook the pasta according to the packet instructions. Drain and keep warm.

3. Stir the chopped basil into the sauce, then stir the sauce into the drained pasta. Sprinkle with a little grated Parmesan cheese (1½ Syns per 1 tbsp), if desired, and a few whole basil leaves before serving.

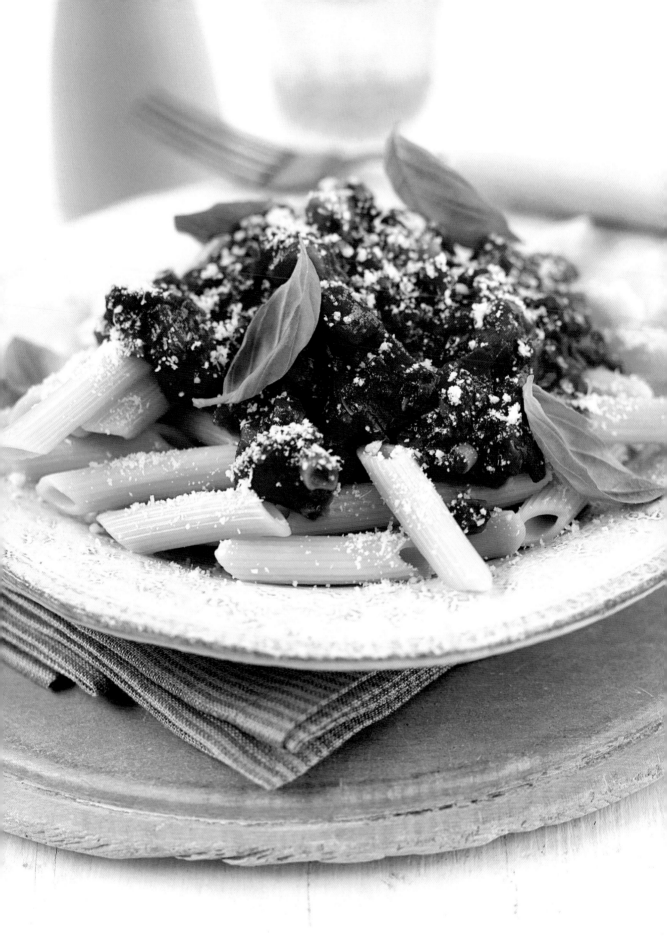

cannelloni

Usually filled with a mixture of ricotta cheese and spinach, this low-Syn and delicious version of the Italian classic uses quark instead.

SERVES 4 ⓥ ❄
WORTH THE EFFORT
Syns per serving
Green: 7
Original: 10½

Preparation time 20 minutes
Cooking time 20–25 minutes

500g/1lb 2oz quark

1 small egg, lightly beaten

200g/7oz canned mushrooms, drained and chopped

300g/11oz cooked spinach, finely chopped

2 tbsp finely chopped basil

4 garlic cloves, peeled and crushed

¼ tsp grated nutmeg

salt and freshly ground black pepper

6 dried lasagne sheets, cooked and drained

500ml/18fl oz passata with herbs and garlic

200g/7oz reduced fat Cheddar cheese, finely grated

1. Preheat the oven to 200°C/Gas 6. Place the quark in a bowl and break it up with a fork. Add the egg, mushrooms, spinach, basil, garlic, nutmeg and seasoning. Mix until well combined.

2. Cut each lasagne sheet in half widthways. Spread 2–3 tbsp of the spinach mixture across the middle of each half, then roll into a tube.

3. Spread a layer of passata in the bottom of an 18 x 25cm/7 x 10in ovenproof dish. Place the filled cannelloni tubes, seam-side down, in a single layer in the dish. Pour the remaining passata over the top and sprinkle with the cheese. Bake in the oven for 20–25 minutes, or until bubbling and lightly golden on top. Serve with a crisp green salad.

risotto primavera

The title of this dish translates as 'spring risotto', and it's aptly named. The creamy rice contains a variety of spring ingredients that impart dazzling colour and flavour.

SERVES 4 Ⓥ ❄

EASY

Syns per serving

Green: Free

Original: 11½

Preparation time 15 minutes

Cooking time about 35 minutes

Fry Light

8–10 spring onions, finely chopped

2 garlic cloves, peeled and finely chopped

4 baby leeks, finely sliced

6 baby courgettes, thinly sliced

6 baby carrots, thinly sliced

250g/9oz Arborio or risotto rice

900ml/32fl oz boiling water or stock made with Vecon

400g/14oz asparagus tips, trimmed

salt and freshly ground black pepper

6 tbsp chopped flat-leaf parsley

To serve

freshly grated Parmesan cheese (optional)

1. Spray a large, non-stick frying pan with Fry Light and place over a medium heat. Add the spring onions, garlic, leeks, courgettes and carrots and stir-fry for 3–4 minutes.

2. Add the rice to the pan and stir-fry for 2–3 minutes. Add a ladleful of the boiling water or stock and cook, stirring, until the liquid has been absorbed. Continue adding the water or stock a ladleful at a time until half of it has been used.

3. Stir in the asparagus, then continue adding the water or stock as before until it is all used up and the rice is creamy and al dente (tender but still retaining a bite). This should take about 20–25 minutes.

4. Remove from the heat, season well and stir in the parsley. Ladle into warmed pasta bowls, sprinkle with grated Parmesan (1½ Syns per 1 tbsp), if desired, and serve immediately

herbed gnocchi

These delicious, Italian-style potato dumplings make a wonderful lunch when served with a rocket salad.

SERVES 4 Ⓥ ✱

WORTH THE EFFORT

Syns per serving
Green: 3½
Original: 11

Preparation time 20 minutes plus chilling
Cooking time about 25 minutes

100g/3½oz mixed fresh herbs (chervil, chives and flat-leaf parsley), finely chopped

800g/1lb 12oz potatoes, peeled, boiled and drained

¼ tsp grated nutmeg

1 small egg, beaten

salt and freshly ground black pepper

2 x 400g cans chopped tomatoes

1 onion, peeled and finely diced

3 garlic cloves, peeled and crushed

2 tbsp finely chopped fresh basil

100g/3½oz reduced fat Cheddar cheese, grated

1. Place the chopped herbs in a bowl with the boiled potatoes, nutmeg and egg. Season well and mash thoroughly. Cover and refrigerate overnight.

2. Preheat the oven to 190°C/Gas 5. Place the tomatoes, onion, garlic and basil in a saucepan and bring to the boil. Cook over a high heat for 6–8 minutes, seasoning well. Spread the mixture in the bottom of a medium, shallow, ovenproof dish and set aside.

3. On a clean work surface, shape the chilled potato mixture into walnut-sized balls or ovals. Place them in a single layer on top of the tomato mixture. Sprinkle the grated cheese over them and bake in the oven for 10 minutes, until hot and bubbling. Serve immediately with a crisp green salad.

veal saltimbocca

Ready in minutes, this Italian favourite makes an ideal after-work supper. It's so good that it *saltimbocca* – 'jumps into the mouth'.

SERVES 4

EASY

Syns per serving
Original: 2
Green: 25½

Preparation time 5 minutes
Cooking time about 10 minutes

8 x 200g/7oz veal escalopes, all visible fat removed

freshly ground black pepper

16 sage leaves

8 very thin slices Parma ham

Fry Light

3 tbsp Marsala or any robust red wine

250ml/9fl oz stock made with Chicken Bovril

1 tbsp chicken gravy granules

To serve

lemon wedges

steamed green beans and carrots

1. Place the escalopes between sheets of cling film and lightly beat them with a meat mallet or rolling pin until about 1cm/½in thick. Remove the cling film, season the veal with black pepper and lay out on a clean work surface. Place 2 sage leaves on each escalope and top with a slice of the Parma ham. Fold each escalope in half, ham-side out, and secure with a cocktail stick.

2. Spray a large, non-stick frying pan with Fry Light and place over a high heat. Add the escalopes and fry on each side for 3–4 minutes, or until just cooked through. Using a slotted spoon, remove from the pan and keep warm.

3. Pour the Marsala or red wine into the pan and cook over a high heat for 30–40 seconds. Add the stock and gravy granules, bring to the boil, then simmer for 4–5 minutes.

4. To serve, place 2 escalopes in the centre of a warmed plate and spoon over the reduced stock mixture. Garnish with lemon wedges and accompany with steamed green beans and carrots.

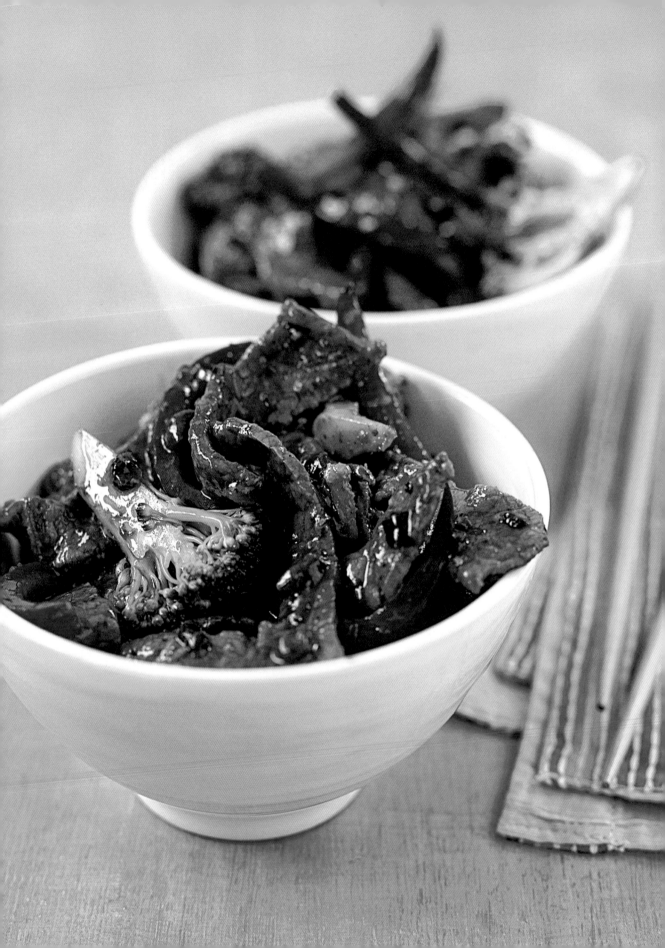

beef
in black bean sauce

This versatile Chinese dish makes a great summer's day lunch when served with a green salad or with Free vegetables of your choice.

SERVES 4 ❋

EASY

Syns per serving
Original: 2½
Green: 10

Preparation time 10 minutes
Cooking time under 15 minutes

450g/1lb lean beef fillet, cut into thin strips

1 tbsp light soy sauce

1 tbsp Shaoxing rice wine or dry sherry

1 tsp salt

1 tsp sugar

1 tsp sesame oil

2 tsp cornflour

1 tbsp finely chopped fresh root ginger

1 tbsp coarsely chopped garlic

2 tbsp finely chopped shallots

1 red pepper, deseeded and cut into thin strips

200g broccoli florets, blanched

6 tbsp finely chopped spring onions

100ml/3½fl oz Blue Dragon black bean sauce

150ml/5fl oz stock made with Beef Bovril

1. Put the beef in a bowl, add the soy sauce, rice wine or sherry, salt, sugar, sesame oil and cornflour and mix together.

2. Place a wok over a high heat. When it is very hot and slightly smoking, add the beef mixture and stir-fry for 2 minutes. Add the ginger, garlic, shallots, red pepper, broccoli, spring onions and black bean sauce and stir-fry for 2 minutes.

3. Pour in the stock, bring the mixture to the boil, then reduce the heat, cover and simmer for 3 minutes, or until the beef is cooked. Serve immediately.

sweet and sour chicken

This Chinese dish brings together lots of contrasting flavours and textures that make for a very satisfying meal.

SERVES 4 ❅

EASY

Syns per serving
Original: 2½
Green: 8½

Preparation time 15 minutes
Cooking time under 20 minutes

450g/1lb chicken breast fillets, skinless and cut into bite-sized pieces

1 egg white

4 tbsp water

175g/6oz canned water chestnuts, drained and coarsely chopped

2 tbsp light soy sauce

1 tbsp dark soy sauce

2 tbsp Shaoxing rice wine or dry sherry

1 tbsp artificial sweetener

2 tsp salt

2 tsp freshly ground black pepper

110g/4oz green pepper, deseeded and cut into 2.5cm/1in pieces

110g/4oz red pepper, deseeded and cut into 2.5cm/1in pieces

110g/4oz carrots, peeled and thinly sliced on the diagonal

1 tbsp cornflour

Fry Light

50g/2oz spring onions (about 4), cut into 2.5cm/1in pieces

For the sauce

150ml/5fl oz stock made with Chicken Bovril

1 tbsp light soy sauce

2 tsp dark soy sauce

1 tsp sesame oil

2 tbsp Chinese white rice vinegar or cider vinegar

1 tbsp artificial sweetener

2 tbsp passata

2 tsp cornflour, blended to a paste with 1 tbsp water

To serve

spring onion curls (optional)

1. Put the chicken, egg white and water in a bowl and mix together using your hands. Add the water chestnuts, the light and dark soy sauces, rice wine, sweetener, salt and pepper and mix well.

2. Bring a pan of water to the boil and blanch the peppers and carrots for 4 minutes, until just tender. Drain and set aside.

3. Sprinkle the chicken with the cornflour and mix together. Spray a large, non-stick wok with Fry Light and place over a medium heat. Add the chicken and stir-fry until cooked through. Remove with a slotted spoon and drain on kitchen paper.

4. Place all the sauce ingredients, except the cornflour paste, in a large saucepan and bring to the boil. Add the peppers, carrots and spring onions and mix well. Stir in the cornflour paste, cook for 2 minutes, then lower the heat to a simmer. Add the chicken to the sauce and cook gently for 4–5 minutes. Serve garnished with spring onion curls, if using.

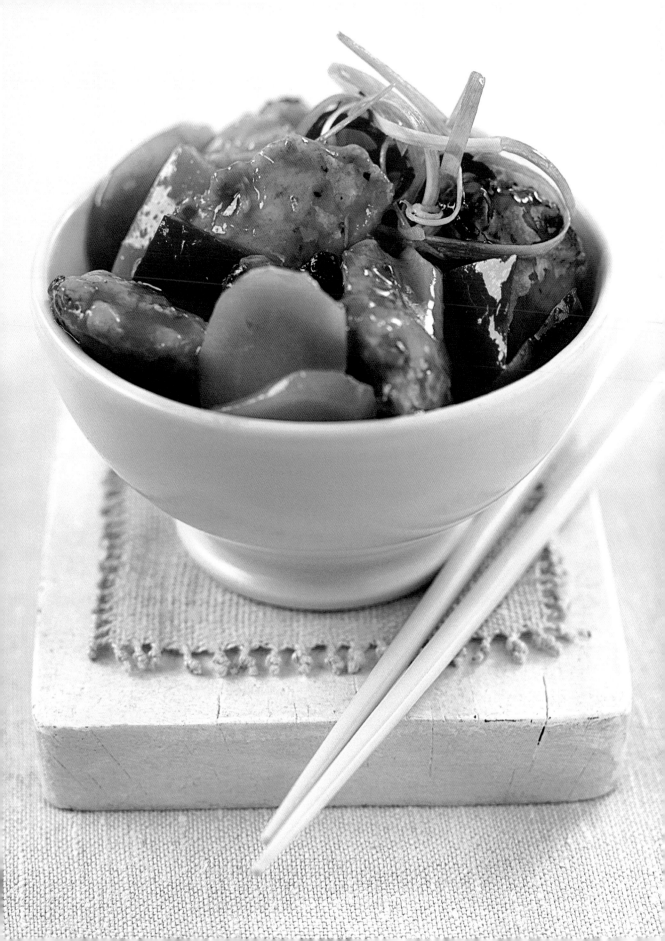

peking duck
in lettuce wraps

Crisp lettuce leaves make a delicious alternative to Chinese pancakes. These wraps are perfect for entertaining as your guests can assemble their own at the table.

SERVES 4

EASY

Syns per serving
Original: 1½
Green: 13

Preparation time 20 minutes
Cooking time about 10 minutes

4 x 175g/6oz duck breasts, skinless

6 tsp Chinese five-spice powder

1 tbsp Szechuan peppercorns, coarsely ground

1 tsp ground star anise

1 tsp sesame oil

8 large iceberg lettuce leaves

2 tbsp hoisin sauce

1 bunch spring onions, finely shredded

½ cucumber, halved lengthways, deseeded and cut into matchsticks

1. Preheat the oven to 180°C/Gas 4. Cut the duck into thick strips and place in a ceramic bowl. Mix together the five-spice powder, ground peppercorns, star anise and sesame oil and sprinkle over the duck.

2. Place a frying pan or wok over a high heat. When hot, add the duck and stir-fry for 10 minutes, until browned and thoroughly cooked.

3. Using two forks, roughly shred the duck pieces and place in a warmed dish.

4. Place 2 lettuce leaves on each serving plate. Spoon a little hoisin sauce into the centre of each leaf, then top with the spring onions, cucumber and shredded duck. Roll each leaf around the filling and serve immediately.

egg fried rice

If you wish, extra finely diced vegetables can be added to the basic rice mixture to make a substantial meal. Carrots, green beans and peppers work really well.

SERVES 4 Ⓥ ❋

EASY

Syns per serving

Green: Free

Original: 4½

Preparation time 10 minutes

Cooking time under 10 minutes

1 egg

Fry Light

200g/7oz cooked long grain rice, left to go cold

100g/3½oz frozen peas, defrosted

4 spring onions, finely chopped

2–3 tsp soy sauce

ground white pepper

1. Beat the egg with 1 tablespoon of water and set aside.

2. Spray a non-stick wok or large frying pan with Fry Light and place over a high heat. When almost smoking, add the rice and stir-fry for about 3–4 minutes, until completely heated through.

3. Add the peas and spring onions. Stir-fry for about 3 minutes, turning the rice constantly around the pan. Season with the soy sauce and white pepper, then push to one side of the pan.

4. Pour the beaten egg mixture into the cleared side of the pan and leave for about 10 seconds so that it begins to set. Using a chopstick, briskly swirl the egg around to break it up, then toss to mix with the rice. Stir-fry the mixture for a further minute and serve immediately.

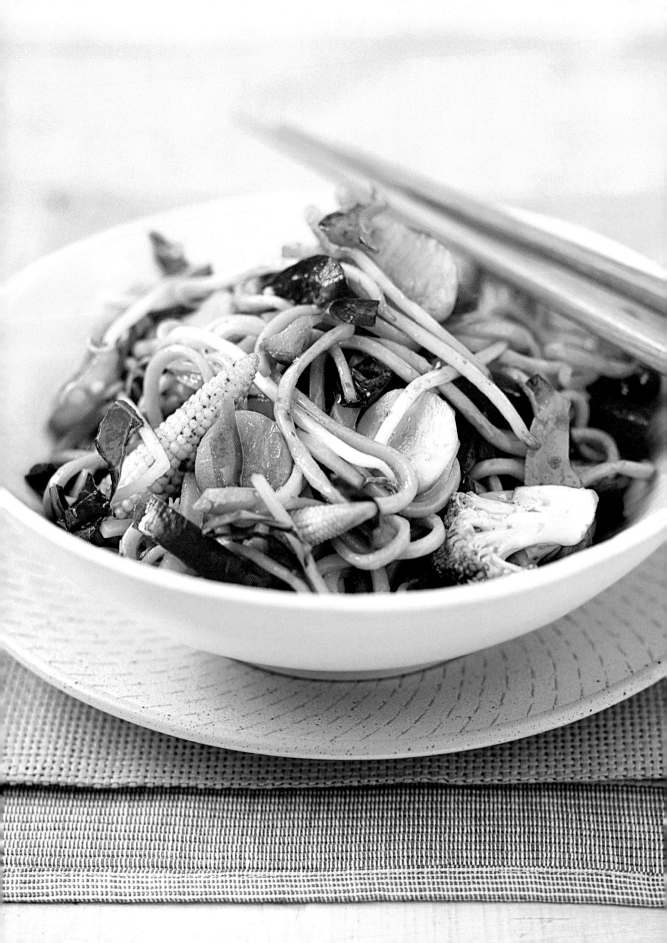

chinese
vegetable stir-fry

This quick and easy stir-fry is a great family favourite and can be made with almost any fresh vegetables you have at hand.

SERVES 4 ⓥ ❋

EASY

Syns per serving
Green: Free
Original: 12½

Preparation time 5 minutes
Cooking time about 10 minutes

1 x 250g packet dried medium egg noodles

Fry Light

10 spring onions, cut into 4cm/1½in lengths

2 garlic cloves, peeled and crushed

1 tsp finely grated fresh root ginger

200g/7oz baby sweetcorn

1 red pepper, deseeded and finely sliced

50g/2oz bean sprouts

6–8 tbsp dark soy sauce

1. Boil the noodles according to the packet instructions.

2. Meanwhile, spray a large, non-stick wok with Fry Light and place over a high heat. Add the spring onions, garlic, ginger, sweetcorn, red pepper and bean sprouts and stir-fry over a high heat for 6–8 minutes.

3. Drain the cooked noodles and add to the wok with the soy sauce. Toss well and stir-fry for 1–2 minutes. Serve hot in warmed bowls.

thai green vegetable curry

The vegetables for this creamy Thai curry can be varied endlessly according to what you have in store, making it very versatile.

SERVES 4 ⓥ ❄
EASY
Syns per serving
Original: 1
Green: 1

Preparation time 20 minutes
Cooking time about 15 minutes

Fry Light
400ml/14fl oz water or stock made with Vecon
6 tbsp Blue Dragon light coconut milk
200g/7oz carrots, peeled and cut into matchsticks

200g/7oz baby sweetcorn, trimmed and halved lengthways
200g/7oz green beans, trimmed and halved
1 red pepper, deseeded and thinly sliced
salt and freshly ground black pepper

For the curry paste
6 shallots, peeled and finely chopped
50g/2oz fresh coriander, roughly chopped
1–2 green chillies, deseeded and roughly chopped

2 garlic cloves, peeled and chopped
1 tsp finely grated fresh root ginger
1 tbsp finely chopped lemongrass
3 tsp ground cumin
1 tsp ground coriander
200ml/7fl oz water

To serve
sweet basil leaves
red chilli slivers
Thai jasmine rice

1. Start by making the curry paste. Place all the ingredients in a blender and process until smooth.

2. Spray a large frying pan with Fry Light and place over a high heat. Add the curry paste and stir-fry for 2–3 minutes.

3. Add the water or stock, coconut milk and vegetables and bring to the boil. Reduce the heat to low and cook gently for 8–10 minutes, or until the vegetables are just tender. Season well and garnish with the basil leaves and chilli before serving. Accompany with Thai jasmine rice (Free on Green; 2 Syns per 25g/1oz cooked on Original).

fragrant carrot and mushroom pilau rice

The key feature of pilaus is that the rice is fried before being cooked in stock. Almost any ingredients you fancy can be added to that savoury base.

SERVES 4 ⓥ ❋

WORTH THE EFFORT

Syns per serving

Green: Free

Original: 9

Preparation time 10 minutes

Cooking time under 30 minutes, plus standing

Fry Light

1 onion, peeled and finely chopped

1 tsp finely grated fresh root ginger

2 garlic cloves, peeled and crushed

½ tsp ground turmeric

1 tbsp mild curry powder

2 cloves

2 carrots, peeled and finely chopped

300g/11oz button mushrooms, halved or quartered

200g/7oz Basmati rice

salt

500ml/18fl oz boiling water

a handful of chopped coriander leaves

1. Spray a non-stick saucepan with Fry Light and place over a medium heat. Add the onion and stir-fry for 5–6 minutes, until softened and lightly browned.

2. Add the ginger, garlic, turmeric, curry powder and cloves and stir-fry for 2–3 minutes. Stir in the vegetables and cook for 2–3 minutes. Add the rice and stir-fry for 2–3 minutes. Season well with salt.

3. Pour the water into the pan and return to the boil. Cover tightly, reduce the heat to very low and leave to cook undisturbed for 12–15 minutes. Remove from the heat and allow to stand, again undisturbed, for 15 minutes.

4. Before serving, fluff up the grains of rice with a fork and stir in the coriander.

vegetable
pad thai

This substantial and colourful noodle and vegetable stir-fry makes a fabulous Green day main course that will have everyone wanting more.

SERVES 4 ⓥ

EASY

Syns per serving
Green: Free
Original: 12½

Preparation time 15 minutes
Cooking time under 15 minutes

2 garlic cloves, peeled and crushed

2 tsp finely grated fresh root ginger

1–2 red chillies, deseeded and finely chopped

6 spring onions, cut into 2.5cm/1in lengths

75ml/3fl oz water or stock made with Vecon

3 tbsp dark soy sauce

¼ tsp artificial sweetener (optional)

2 carrots, peeled and cut into fine matchsticks

200g/7oz mangetout, thinly sliced

250g/9oz bean sprouts

250g/9oz dried flat medium rice noodles

1 egg, lightly beaten

To serve

sliced spring onion

freshly chopped coriander

freshly squeezed lime juice

1. Place the garlic, ginger, chillies, spring onions, water or stock, soy sauce and sweetener (if using) in a large, non-stick frying pan. Heat gently for 4–5 minutes.

2. Turn the heat to high and add the vegetables. Stir-fry for 4–5 minutes, until the vegetables are just tender.

3. Prepare the noodles according to the packet instructions, drain and add to the vegetable mixture in the frying pan over a high heat. Drizzle over the beaten egg, mix well and cook for 1–2 minutes, until the egg is just cooked through. Before serving, sprinkle over the spring onion, coriander and lime juice.

spinach dhal

This satisfying lentil dish is a healthy and delicious way to warm up on a cold winter's day.

SERVES 4 Ⓥ ❄

EASY

Syns per serving
Green: Free
Original: 6½

Preparation time 10 minutes
Cooking time about 30 minutes

Fry Light

2 onions, peeled and finely chopped

4 garlic cloves, peeled and finely chopped

1 red chilli, deseeded and finely sliced

1 tsp finely grated fresh root ginger

1 tbsp cumin seeds

1 tbsp black mustard seeds

2 tbsp mild curry powder

175g/6oz dried red split lentils

600ml/22fl oz water

2 red peppers, deseeded and roughly chopped

200g/7oz baby spinach leaves, roughly chopped

salt

8–10 tbsp finely chopped coriander

To serve

steamed basmati rice (optional)

1. Spray a medium saucepan with Fry Light and place over a medium heat. Add the onions and stir-fry for 1–2 minutes. Reduce the heat and stir in the garlic, chilli, ginger, cumin seeds, mustard seeds and curry powder. Stir-fry for 1–2 minutes.

2. Add the lentils and water. Bring to the boil, add the peppers and spinach and reduce the heat to low. Cover and simmer gently, stirring occasionally, for 15–20 minutes, until the mixture is thick and the lentils are just tender.

3. Season the dhal with salt, then remove from the heat and stir in the chopped coriander. Serve immediately over steamed basmati rice (Free on Green; 2 Syns per 25g/1oz on Original), if desired.

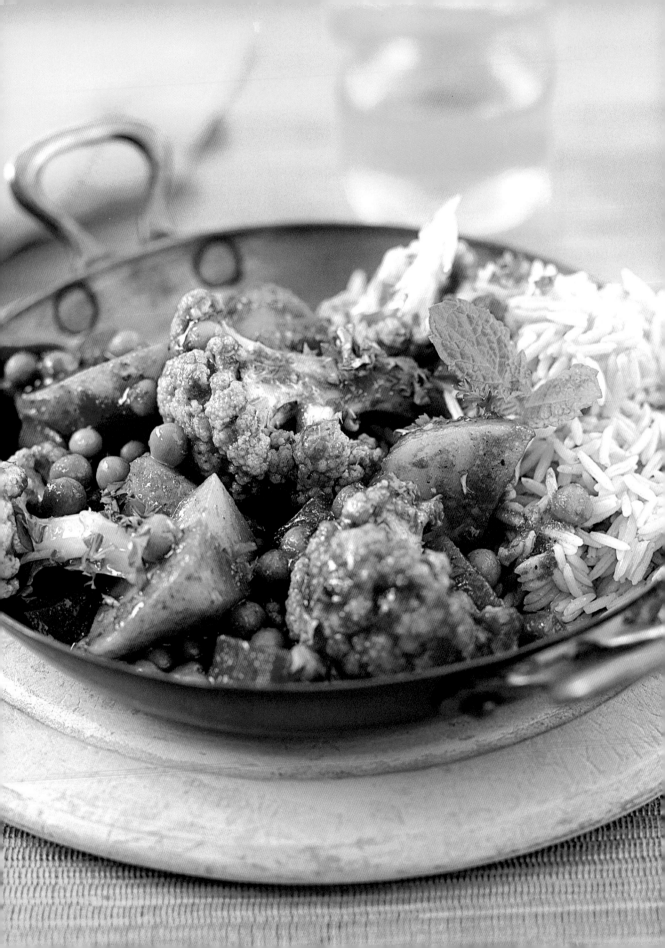

aloo gobi

This Indian vegetarian dish of cauliflower and potato in a spiced tomato sauce is so tasty that even meat-eaters love it.

SERVES 4 ⓥ ❋

EASY

Syns per serving
Green: Free
Original: 7½

Preparation time 15 minutes
Cooking time under 30 minutes

Fry Light

2 onions, peeled and finely chopped

2 tsp garlic granules

2 tsp ground ginger

2 tbsp mild curry powder

500g/1lb 2oz potatoes, peeled and cut into small bite-sized pieces

300g/11oz cauliflower florets

1 red pepper, deseeded and cut into bite-sized pieces

300g/11oz frozen peas

500ml/18fl oz passata

200ml/7fl oz water

1 tsp artificial sweetener

To serve

a large handful of chopped mint and coriander

steamed basmati rice (optional)

1. Spray a large, non-stick frying pan with Fry Light and place over a medium heat. Add the onions and stir-fry for 2–3 minutes.

2. Add the garlic granules, ginger and curry powder and stir-fry for 20–30 seconds. Add the potatoes, cauliflower, red pepper and peas and stir-fry for 2–3 minutes.

3. Stir in the passata, water and sweetener and bring to the boil. Cover, reduce the heat to medium and cook, stirring now and again, for 15–20 minutes, or until the vegetables are tender. Serve garnished with chopped mint and coriander, and with steamed basmati rice (Free on Green; 2 Syns per 25g/1oz cooked on Original), if desired.

lamb
rogan josh

Seasoned with fragrant spices, this slow-cooked curry produces lamb that
is meltingly tender – a treat for all the senses.

SERVES 4 ✽

EASY

Syns per serving

Original: Free

Green: 15

Preparation time 15 minutes

Cooking time about 2½ hours

Fry Light

800g/1lb 12oz lamb shoulder,
boneless and cut into large
bite-sized pieces

2 large onions, peeled, halved
and thickly sliced

4 garlic cloves, peeled and
crushed

2 tsp finely grated fresh root
ginger

2 sticks cinnamon

4 tsp paprika

2 tsp crushed cardamom
seeds

4 tbsp medium curry powder

1 x 400g can chopped
tomatoes

1 tsp artificial sweetener

600ml/22fl oz stock made with
Chicken Bovril

600g/1lb 6oz swede, peeled
and cut into large pieces

salt and freshly ground black
pepper

To serve

freshly chopped coriander

very low fat natural yogurt,
whisked

1. Spray a large, heavy-based casserole with Fry Light and cook
   the lamb, in batches, for 3–4 minutes, until browned. Remove
   with a slotted spoon and set aside.

2. Spray the casserole again and add the onions. Cook over a
   medium heat for 10–12 minutes, stirring often, until soft and
   lightly browned.

3. Add the garlic, ginger, cinnamon, paprika and cardamom seeds
   and stir-fry for 1–2 minutes. Mix in the curry powder. Return
   lamb to the casserole and stir-fry for a further 2–3 minutes. Stir
   in the tomatoes, sweetener, stock and swede. Season well and
   bring to the boil.

4. Reduce the heat to very low (using a heat diffuser if possible)
   and cover tightly. Simmer gently for 2 hours, or until the lamb is
   meltingly tender. Serve garnished with chopped coriander and
   drizzled with yogurt.

classic chicken curry

If you like a more fiery curry, increase the amount of green chilli to suit your palate, or simply leave the seeds in when you add it.

SERVES 4 ❋

EASY

Syns per serving
Original: Free
Green: 11

Preparation time 10 minutes
Cooking time about 50 minutes

Fry Light

1 onion, peeled and finely chopped

1 green chilli, deseeded and finely chopped or sliced

2 tsp finely grated garlic

2 tsp finely grated fresh root ginger

800g/1lb 12oz chicken breasts or thighs, skinless and boneless, cut into bite-sized pieces

3–4 tbsp mild or medium curry powder

1 x 400g can chopped tomatoes

1 tsp artificial sweetener

100ml/3½fl oz stock made with Chicken Bovril

salt and freshly ground black pepper

a large handful of freshly chopped coriander and mint

1. Spray a large, non-stick frying pan with Fry Light and place over a medium heat. When hot, add the onion, chilli, garlic and ginger and stir-fry for 4–5 minutes. Add the chicken and curry powder, mix well and stir-fry for 3–4 minutes.

2. Add the tomatoes, sweetener and stock to the pan and bring to the boil. Cover, lower the heat and cook gently for 30–35 minutes, or until the chicken is cooked through and tender.

3. Remove the pan from the heat, season well and stir in the chopped herbs. Serve immediately.

chicken tikka

This restaurant classic can be prepared and marinated up to a day in advance and quickly cooked whenever you're ready. Accompany with a cucumber raita, made by grating half a cucumber into 250g/9oz very low fat natural yogurt, seasoning to taste and sprinkling with a little paprika.

SERVES 4 ❅

EASY

Syns per serving
Original: Free
Green: 9½

Preparation time 15 minutes
plus marinating
Cooking time 12–15 minutes

700g/1lb 8oz chicken breast fillets, skinless, cut into bite-sized pieces

2 red peppers, deseeded and cut into 2.5cm/1in pieces

2 small red onions, peeled and cut into quarters

2–3 tbsp tikka masala powder or medium-hot curry powder

2 tbsp passata

2 garlic cloves, peeled and crushed

2 tsp finely grated fresh root ginger

150g/5oz very low fat natural yogurt

salt and freshly ground black pepper

To serve
coriander leaves
cucumber raita
lime wedges

1. Place the chicken in a ceramic bowl with the red peppers and red onion. Put the tikka masala powder, passata, garlic, ginger and yogurt in a separate bowl and mix together. Season, then pour this marinade over the chicken mixture. Stir well, cover and refrigerate for 2–3 hours, or overnight if time permits.

2. Preheat the grill to medium high. Meanwhile, thread the chicken and vegetables onto 8 metal skewers. Grill the kebabs, turning once or twice, for 12–15 minutes, or until cooked through and lightly charred at the edges.

3. Serve immediately, garnished with coriander and accompanied by cucumber raita and wedges of lime.

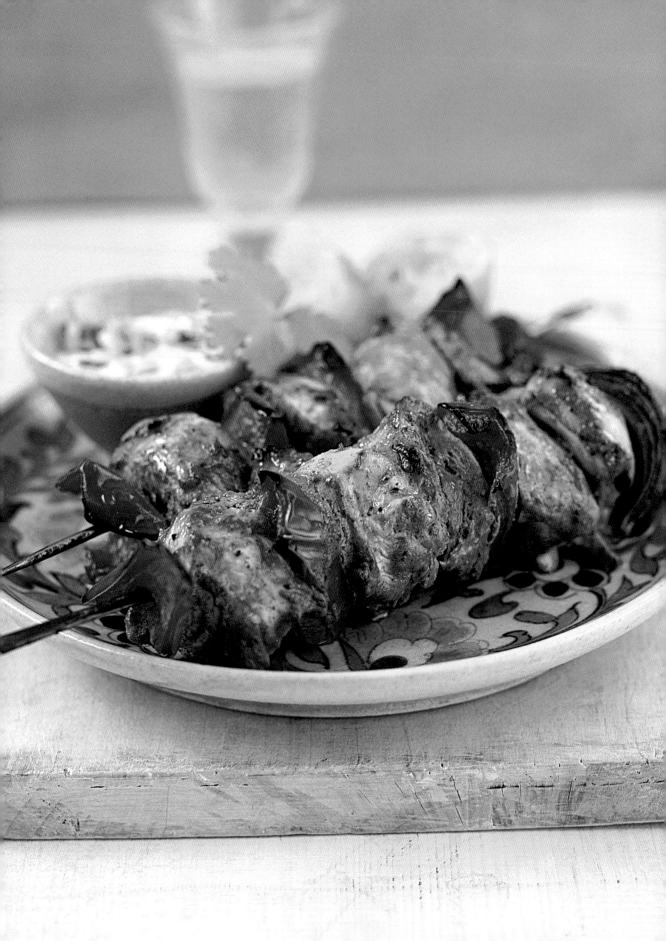

prawn curry

If you have access to fresh prawns, use them instead of the cooked ones listed below: just peel and devein them before adding to the pan, and cook for 3–4 minutes, or until they turn pink and are cooked through.

SERVES 4

EASY

Syns per serving
Original: Free
Green: 10

Preparation time 5 minutes
Cooking time about 20 minutes

2 tbsp mild or medium curry powder

4 garlic cloves, peeled and crushed

2 tsp finely grated fresh root ginger

1 x 400g can chopped tomatoes

½ tsp artificial sweetener

800g/1lb 12oz cooked tiger prawns

200g/7oz very low fat natural yogurt

salt and freshly ground black pepper

To serve
freshly chopped coriander

1. Place the curry powder, garlic, ginger, tomatoes and sweetener in a saucepan and bring to the boil. Cover, reduce the heat and simmer gently for 8–10 minutes.

2. Add the prawns and cook for 2–3 minutes, or until warmed through. Remove from the heat and stir in the yogurt. Season well and serve immediately, garnished with the coriander.

hungarian goulash

A touch of paprika gives an intriguing and smoky flavour to this classic Hungarian stew, which really benefits from long, slow simmering.

SERVES 4 ❀

EASY

Syns per serving
Original: Free
Green: 14

Preparation time 15–20 minutes
Cooking time 2–2½ hours

Fry Light

12 shallots, peeled and halved

2 garlic cloves, peeled and finely chopped

2 carrots, peeled and cut into bite-sized pieces

1 bay leaf

100g/3½oz canned lean ham, cut into small bite-sized cubes

2 tsp paprika

800g/1lb 12oz lean beef fillet, cut into bite-sized pieces

2 red peppers, deseeded and cut into bite-sized pieces

1 x 400g can chopped tomatoes

200ml/7fl oz stock made with Beef Bovril

salt and freshly ground black pepper

To serve

freshly chopped parsley

1. Spray a large, non-stick frying pan with Fry Light and place over a medium heat. Add the shallots and stir-fry for 2–3 minutes, until brown. Add the garlic, carrots and bay leaf and stir-fry for 2–3 minutes.

2. Add the ham, paprika, beef and red peppers and stir-fry for 6–8 minutes.

3. Add the tomatoes and stock and bring to the boil. Season well, then cover tightly and cook gently, stirring occasionally, for 1½–2 hours, or until the beef is tender. Discard the bay leaf and stir in the chopped parsley before serving.

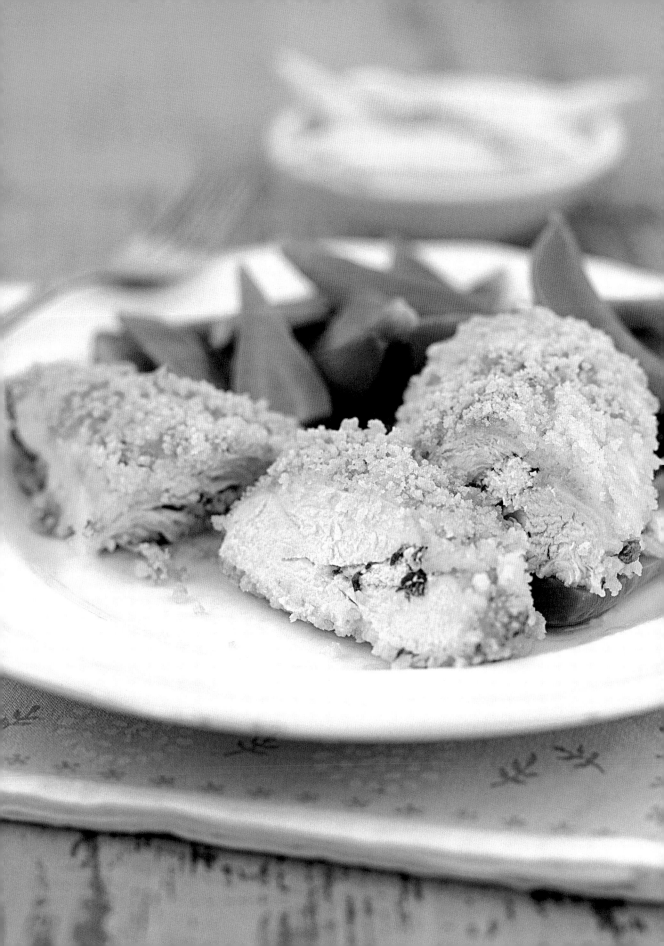

chicken kiev

Traditional chicken Kiev is filled with luscious garlic butter, but our version offers a lighter option, using quark. It turns ordinary chicken breasts into an impressive restaurant-style meal.

SERVES 4
WORTH THE EFFORT
Syns per serving
Original: 4½
Green: 12

Preparation time 10 minutes
Cooking time about 20 minutes

4 large chicken breast fillets, skinless
3 medium eggs, beaten
100g/3½oz fine, dry wholemeal breadcrumbs
Fry Light

For the stuffing
1 tbsp very finely chopped spring onions
4 garlic cloves, peeled and crushed
a small handful of flat-leaf parsley, finely chopped
2 tbsp finely chopped tarragon
50g/2oz quark
salt and freshly ground black pepper

To serve
steamed vegetables (carrots, mangetout, baby sweetcorn)

1. Start by making the stuffing. Place all the ingredients in a bowl, season generously with pepper and a little salt and beat until completely combined. Tip onto a sheet of cling film and roll into a log. Chill until required. (This part of the recipe can be made up to 3 days in advance if refrigerated, or up to 1 month if frozen.)

2. Make an incision along the side of each chicken fillet, cutting halfway into the meat to make a pocket (it is essential not to cut all the way through). Lay a piece of cling film over each fillet and beat lightly with a meat mallet or rolling pin to flatten slightly.

3. Divide the stuffing mixture into 4 equal pieces and shape into flattish ovals. Push these ovals into the chicken pockets.

4. Tip the eggs and breadcrumbs into separate shallow containers. Dip each breast in the egg, then in the breadcrumbs, the aim being to coat them completely. Set aside.

5. Preheat the oven to 200°C/Gas 6. Spray the chicken pieces with Fry Light and place in a non-stick roasting tin. Bake in the oven for 20 minutes, or until the Kievs are lightly golden and cooked through. Serve immediately with steamed vegetables.

lamb souvlaki

These Greek lamb skewers are great for a mid-week supper as they are quick to cook and really delicious. Marinate the lamb the night before so that the meal can be ready in minutes when you get home.

SERVES 4 ❋

EASY

Syns per serving
Original: Free
Green: 15

Preparation time 15 minutes
plus marinating
Cooking time about 10 minutes

800g/1lb 12oz lean lamb leg steaks, cut into cubes

juice and finely grated zest of 3 lemons

2 tbsp dried oregano

2 tbsp dried mint

3 garlic cloves, peeled and crushed

salt and freshly ground black pepper

2 onions, peeled and cut into large pieces

1 red pepper, deseeded and cut into large pieces

1 yellow pepper, deseeded and cut into large pieces

To serve
lettuce and tomato salad

1. Place the lamb in a shallow, ceramic bowl. Put the lemon juice and zest, oregano, mint and garlic in a separate bowl, mix well, then pour over the lamb. Season well and leave to marinate in the fridge for 6–8 hours, or overnight if time permits.

2. Preheat the grill to medium hot. Thread the lamb, onion and pepper pieces alternately on 8 skewers. Grill the kebabs for 4–5 minutes on each side, or until cooked to your liking. Serve the souvlaki with a lettuce and tomato salad.

vegetable stroganoff

Russian in origin, this hearty vegetable 'stew' is a great way to cook mushrooms and peppers, and makes a filling lunch or dinner when served with rice.

SERVES 4 ⓥ

EASY

Syns per serving
Original: Free
Green: Free

Preparation time 10 minutes
Cooking time under 30 minutes

400ml/14fl oz passata with herbs

150ml/5fl oz water or stock made with Vecon

2 onions, peeled and finely chopped

2 garlic cloves, peeled and crushed

2 red peppers, deseeded and cut into bite-sized pieces

500g/1lb 2oz button mushrooms, halved

2 tsp dried mixed herbs

3 tbsp finely chopped chives

salt and freshly ground black pepper

300g/11oz very low fat natural fromage frais

To serve

freshly chopped mixed herbs

boiled rice (optional)

1. Place a large, non-stick frying pan over a high heat. Add the passata, water or stock, onions, garlic, peppers, mushrooms, dried herbs and chives. Season well and bring to the boil. Reduce the heat to medium, then cover and cook for 15–20 minutes.

2. Remove the pan from the heat, stir in the fromage frais and garnish with the chopped herbs. Serve with boiled rice (Free on Green; 2 Syns per 25g/1oz cooked on Original), if desired.

vegetable tagine

Flavoured with cumin, cinnamon, ginger and coriander, this earthy Moroccan vegetable dish is best served over freshly made couscous.

SERVES 4 ⓥ ❄

EASY

Syns per serving
Original: Free
Green: Free

Preparation time 15 minutes
Cooking time about 1 hour

1 large onion, peeled and finely chopped

2 garlic cloves, peeled and crushed

1 tsp finely grated fresh root ginger

2 tsp ground cumin

1 tsp ground coriander

2 tsp ground cinnamon

1 tsp ground turmeric

1 tsp dried chilli flakes

1 x 400g can chopped tomatoes

½ tsp artificial sweetener

250ml/9fl oz water or stock made with Vecon

2 carrots, peeled and cut into bite-sized pieces

200g/7oz baby courgettes, cut into 2.5cm/1in slices

250g/9oz baby aubergines, halved lengthways

200g/7oz baby turnips, trimmed and scrubbed

salt and freshly ground black pepper

To serve

freshly chopped coriander

1. Place a medium non-stick frying pan over a medium heat. Add the onion and stir-fry for 4–5 minutes. Add the garlic, ginger, cumin, coriander, cinnamon, turmeric, chilli flakes, tomatoes, sweetener and water or stock. Bring to the boil, reduce the heat to low, then cover and simmer for 25 minutes.

2. Stir in the vegetables and cook over a medium heat for 20–25 minutes, or until the vegetables are cooked through and tender. Season well and garnish with chopped coriander before serving.

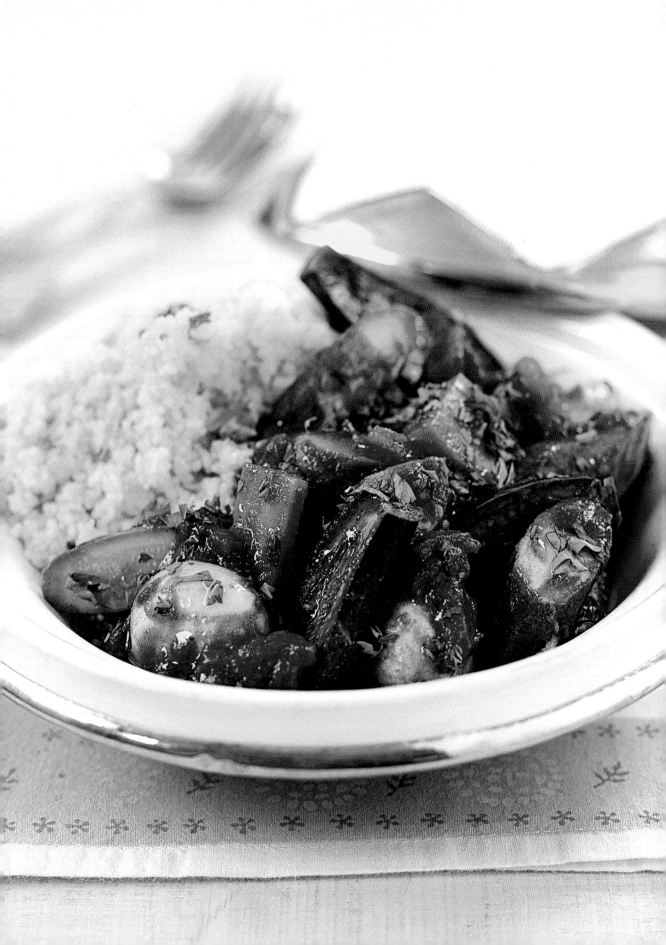

herbed falafels
with cucumber tzatziki

This delicious Middle Eastern mezze dish needs lengthy chilling before cooking, but the result is well worth a little forward planning.

SERVES 4 Ⓥ ❄

EASY

Syns per serving

Green: 4

Original: 16

Preparation time 25 minutes plus chilling

Cooking time 8–10 minutes

800g/1lb 12oz canned chickpeas, rinsed and drained

1 large onion, peeled and finely chopped

12 tbsp finely chopped parsley

15 tbsp finely chopped coriander

4 spring onions, finely chopped

1 tsp baking powder

1 tsp bicarbonate of soda

2 garlic cloves, peeled and crushed

2 tsp ground coriander

2 tsp ground cumin

1 tsp chilli powder

breadcrumbs made from 6 slices of Nimble bread

1 egg, lightly beaten

salt and freshly ground black pepper

Fry Light

For the cucumber tzatziki

½ cucumber, finely diced

5 tbsp finely chopped fresh mint

200g/7oz very low fat natural yogurt

juice of ½ lemon

To serve

lettuce leaves

1. Place all the main ingredients, apart from the Fry Light and lettuce, in a food processor, season well and blend until coarsely puréed. Transfer to a large bowl and mix well with your hands. Cover and refrigerate for 8–10 hours, or overnight if time permits.

2. When ready to cook, preheat the oven to 200°C/Gas 6. Divide the falafel mixture into 12 pieces and shape each one into a flat patty. Place on a non-stick baking sheet lined with baking parchment, spray with Fry Light and bake for 8–10 minutes, or until golden brown. Remove from the oven and set aside.

3. Meanwhile, combine all the tzatziki ingredients in a bowl and season well. Serve the falafels on lettuce leaves with the tzatziki.

spanish-style garlic cauliflower

Typically found in the Navarra and Rioja regions of Spain, this simple but aromatic dish transforms the humble cauliflower into something fresh and exciting. This recipe would work equally well with broccoli.

SERVES 4 ⓥ ❀

EASY

Syns per serving
Original: Free
Green: Free

Preparation time under 10 minutes

Cooking time under 15 minutes

800g/1lb 12oz cauliflower florets, broken into bite-sized pieces

Fry Light

3 garlic cloves, peeled and finely chopped

2 tbsp white wine vinegar

1 tbsp pimenton or mild paprika

salt and freshly ground black pepper

To serve
finely chopped parsley

1. Bring a large saucepan of lightly salted water to the boil. Add the cauliflower, bring back to the boil and cook for 6–8 minutes. Drain thoroughly and set aside.

2. Spray a large, non-stick frying pan with Fry Light and place over a moderate heat. Add the garlic and stir-fry for 1–2 minutes. Add the cauliflower, vinegar and pimenton or paprika and season well. Stir-fry over a high heat for 3–4 minutes. Transfer the mixture to a serving dish, sprinkle over the chopped parsley and serve immediately.

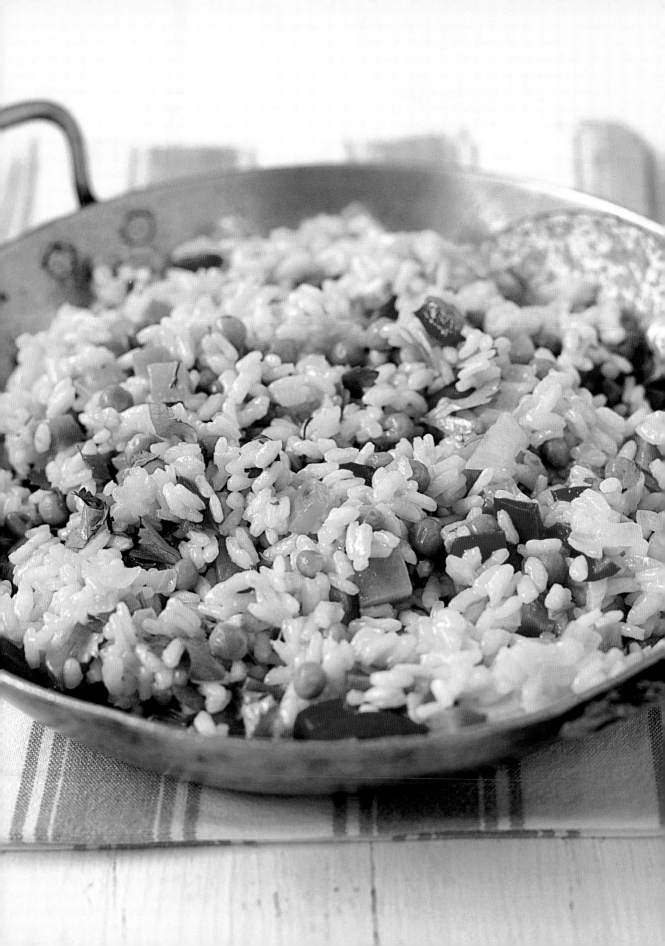

vegetable
paella

Traditional paella contains chicken and seafood, but our version uses a colourful mixture of vegetables instead. Saffron and smoked paprika add a wonderfully exotic flavour to this substantial rice dish.

SERVES 4 Ⓥ ❄
EASY
Syns per serving
Green: Free
Original: 31½

Preparation time 15 minutes
Cooking time under 45 minutes
plus standing

Fry Light

2 medium onions, peeled and finely chopped

4 garlic cloves, peeled and chopped

2 red peppers, deseeded and finely chopped

2 carrots, peeled and cut into 1cm/½in pieces

700g/1lb 8oz long grain rice

3 tbsp finely chopped flat-leaf parsley

1 bay leaf

2 tbsp sweet smoked paprika

a large pinch of saffron threads

1.5 litres/2½ pints water or stock made with Vecon

100g/3½oz frozen peas

1. Spray a paella pan or a large, non-stick frying pan with Fry Light and fry the onions for 4–5 minutes. Add the garlic, red peppers and carrots and fry for 4–5 minutes. Stir in the rice, parsley, bay leaf, paprika and saffron. Pour in the water or stock and peas, bring to a simmer and cook, uncovered, over a gentle heat for 12–15 minutes.

2. After the first phase of cooking, cover the pan tightly, turn the heat to very low and cook for another 12–15 minutes, until the rice is tender, the vegetables are cooked through and all the liquid has been absorbed. Remove from the heat, discard the bay leaf and allow to stand, covered, for 10 minutes. Fluff up the rice with a fork before serving.

spanish-style
potato tortilla

There are two types of tortilla: in South America and Mexico it is a cornmeal pancake, while in Spain it is an omelette that often contains potatoes. Here we give our take on the Spanish version, which resembles a chunky 'cake' and is ideal picnic fare because it is easily portable and can be eaten without cutlery.

SERVES 4 Ⓥ ❋

EASY

Syns per serving
Green: 2
Original: 5

Preparation time 25 minutes
Cooking time about 25 minutes plus standing

Fry Light

1 onion, peeled and finely chopped

300g/11oz cooked, peeled potatoes, cut into 1cm/½in dice

250g/9oz quark

4 eggs

salt and freshly ground black pepper

50g/2oz reduced fat Cheddar cheese, grated

1. Spray a medium, non-stick frying pan with Fry Light and place over a high heat. Sauté the onion for 1–2 minutes. Add the potatoes and cook for another 2 minutes, or until lightly browned.

2. In a separate bowl, whisk together the quark and eggs, then season to taste. Pour over the potato mixture and sprinkle with the cheese. Cook over a medium-low heat for 12–15 minutes, or until the underside of the tortilla is set.

3. Meanwhile, preheat the grill to medium hot. Place the frying pan under it for 4–5 minutes, or until the top of the tortilla is set and lightly golden. Allow to rest for 5 minutes before cutting into wedges and serving.

chicken fajitas

Fajitas are a Tex-Mex invention, consisting of grilled meat traditionally served in a tortilla (cornmeal pancake). We use lettuce leaves rather than pancakes, and you can substitute any type of lean minced meat for the chicken if you wish.

SERVES 4   ❄ (mince only)
WORTH THE EFFORT
Syns per serving
Original: 6
Green: 6

Preparation time 15 minutes
Cooking time about 40 minutes

Fry Light

1 onion, peeled and finely chopped

350g/12oz extra-lean chicken mince

3 tsp garlic salt

2 tsp ground cumin

1 tsp ground cinnamon

2 tsp paprika

2 green peppers, deseeded and finely diced

1 x 400g can chopped tomatoes

1 tsp artificial sweetener

1 tbsp soy sauce

1 x 400g can red kidney beans, rinsed and drained

salt and freshly ground black pepper

For the Mexican salsa

4 tbsp each of finely chopped avocado, red onion, tomato, cucumber, coriander and mint

juice of 1 lemon

To serve

8 large iceberg lettuce leaves

very low fat natural fromage frais or yogurt

1. Place all the salsa ingredients in a bowl and mix together. Set aside until needed.

2. Spray a large, non-stick frying pan with Fry Light and place over a high heat. Add the onion and mince, stir-fry for 5–6 minutes, then add everything up to and including the kidney beans. Season well and bring to the boil. Reduce the heat, cover and cook gently for 25–30 minutes, stirring occasionally.

3. To serve, divide the lettuce leaves between 4 serving plates and spoon in the mince mixture. Top with some salsa and fromage frais or yogurt, roll up into parcels and eat immediately.

classic new york
bacon and cheeseburger

Take-away burgers are often high in fat, so why not try our healthier alternative? You can make a meal of this 'whopper' burger any night of the week.

SERVES 1

WORTH THE EFFORT

Syns per serving
Original: 11
Green: 35½

Preparation time 15 minutes
Cooking time under 15 minutes

250g/9oz extra-lean beef mince

2 tbsp very finely chopped shallots

1 tsp Worcestershire sauce

1 garlic clove, peeled and crushed

salt and freshly ground black pepper

4 lean bacon rashers

To serve

1 x 50g/2oz wholemeal roll, cut in half

lettuce leaves

tomato slices

2 x Kraft Dairylea Light Cheese Slices

mustard

gherkins (optional)

1. Preheat the grill until very hot. Meanwhile, place the beef, shallots, Worcestershire sauce and garlic in a bowl and mix thoroughly using your fingers. Season well and divide in half. Shape each piece into a flat burger and place on the grill pan with the bacon. Grill for 5–6 minutes on each side, or until the burgers are cooked to your liking and the bacon is crisp. Remove and keep warm.

2. To serve, put one half of the bread roll on a plate and place a lettuce leaf, a tomato slice and 2 grilled rashers on it. Top with a burger and a slice of cheese. Add the remaining rashers, burger and cheese slice, and put the other half of the roll on top. Serve immediately with mustard (½ Syn per 1 tbsp) and gherkins, if desired.

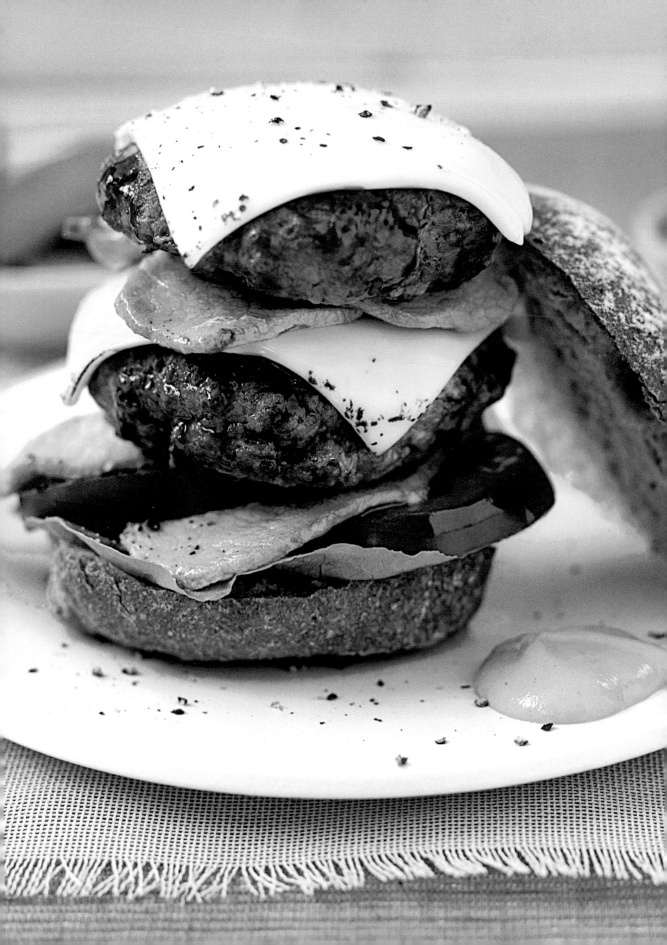

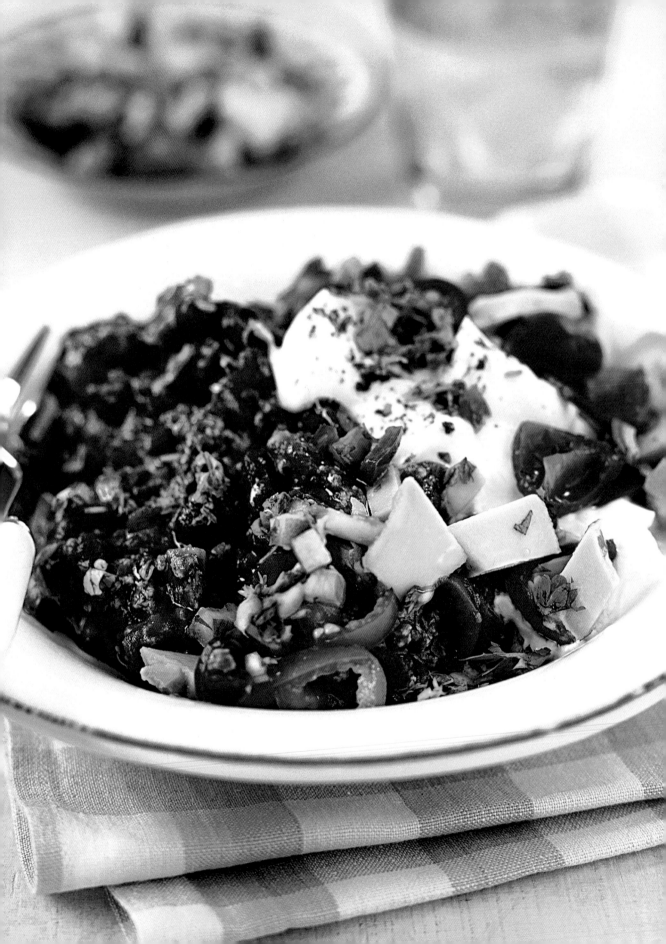

spicy vegetable chilli
with guacamole

The cool and chunky texture of the guacamole complements the robust vegetable chilli perfectly in this economical and healthy dish.

SERVES 4 Ⓥ ❄ (chilli only)

EASY

Syns per serving
Green: 3½
Original: 13½

Preparation time 25–30 minutes
Cooking time about 40 minutes

Fry Light

200g/7oz Quorn mince

1 red onion, peeled, halved and thinly sliced

2 red chillies, deseeded and finely chopped or sliced

2 garlic cloves, peeled and crushed

1 tsp ground ginger

2 tsp ground coriander

2 tsp cumin seeds, crushed

1 carrot, peeled and cut into 1cm/½in dice

2 sticks celery, cut into 1cm/½in dice

1 x 400g can chopped tomatoes

2 x 400g cans red kidney beans, rinsed and drained

salt and freshly ground black pepper

a large handful of coriander leaves, chopped

For the guacamole

1 ripe avocado, stoned, peeled and cut into 1cm/½in dice

1 red onion, peeled and finely diced

2 plum tomatoes, finely diced

1 red chilli, finely chopped

juice of 2 limes

a small handful of coriander leaves, finely chopped

To serve

very low fat natural fromage frais

1. Spray a large, non-stick frying pan with Fry Light and place over a medium heat. Add the Quorn, onion, chillies, garlic, ginger, ground coriander, cumin seeds, carrot and celery and stir-fry for 4–5 minutes.

2. Add the tomatoes and beans, season well and bring to the boil. Reduce the heat and cook gently for 25–30 minutes, stirring often.

3. Meanwhile, make the guacamole. Mix all the ingredients together in a small bowl, season well and set aside until needed.

4. Remove the Quorn mixture from the heat, stir in the chopped coriander and serve immediately, garnished with a little fromage frais and accompanied by the guacamole.

bouillabaisse

Enjoy a taste of southern French cuisine with this wonderfully rich and aromatic fish stew. It's simply bursting with summer flavours.

SERVES 4

EASY

Syns per serving
Original: Free
Green: 25

Preparation time 10–12 minutes
Cooking time about 40 minutes

1 leek, white part only, finely diced

½ fennel bulb, very finely chopped

4 garlic cloves, peeled and thinly sliced

2 tsp fennel seeds

4 ripe tomatoes, roughly chopped

1 tsp artificial sweetener

1.5 litres/2½ pints stock made with Chicken Bovril

1 fresh bouquet garni (2 sprigs of thyme, 1 sprig of parsley and 2 bay leaves, tied with string)

1.5kg/3lb 6oz mixed fish (cod, halibut, red snapper, salmon, etc.), cut into large, even-sized pieces

salt and freshly ground black pepper

cayenne pepper

To serve
finely chopped parsley

1. Place a large, non-stick saucepan over a medium heat. Add all the ingredients up to and including the bouquet garni, and bring to the boil. Cook for 15–20 minutes over a gentle heat.

2. Stir in the fish, bring back to the boil, then reduce the heat and simmer gently for 5–6 minutes, or until the fish has cooked through. Season with salt, pepper and cayenne, then divide the fish between 4 warmed shallow bowls. Strain the soup and ladle it over the fish. Garnish with chopped parsley and serve immediately.

coq au vin

Slow-cooking the chicken with mushrooms, vegetables and red wine in this French-style casserole creates a deliciously satisfying dish that will go down a treat with family or guests.

SERVES 4 ✱

WORTH THE EFFORT

Syns per serving
Original: 1½
Green: 10

Preparation time 20 minutes
Cooking time under 2 hours

Fry Light

4 chicken drumsticks, skinless

4 chicken thighs, skinless

4 lean bacon rashers, chopped

15 pearl or baby button onions, peeled

2 large carrots, peeled and cut into large chunks

1 head of garlic, separated but not peeled

400g/14oz button mushrooms, halved

800ml/28fl oz stock made with Chicken Bovril

1 tbsp Chicken Bovril

200ml/7fl oz red wine

4–5 sprigs of tarragon

4–5 sprigs of thyme

salt and freshly ground black pepper

To serve
freshly chopped parsley

1. Spray a large, non-stick casserole with Fry Light and place over a high heat. Add the chicken pieces and cook until lightly browned on all sides.

2. Add the bacon, onions, carrots, garlic, mushrooms, stock, Bovril, wine and herbs, season well and bring to the boil. Reduce the heat to low, cover very tightly and cook gently for 1½ hours.

3. Check the seasoning and serve immediately in warmed shallow bowls, garnished with the parsley. Accompany with additional Free vegetables of your choice, if wished.

tuna niçoise

This super-healthy salad of fresh tuna with lettuce, tomatoes, green beans and olives is really easy to prepare and perfect for a summer lunch.

SERVES 4

EXTRA EASY

Syns per serving
Original: ½
Green: 12

Preparation time 20 minutes
Cooking time about 4–6 minutes

4 x 175g/6oz fresh tuna steaks

Fry Light

salt and freshly ground black pepper

2 Little Gem lettuces, leaves separated

6 medium tomatoes, quartered

14 black olives, pitted

300g/11oz green beans, trimmed, boiled and cooled

4 hard-boiled eggs, peeled and quartered

6 tbsp fat-free French-style salad dressing

1. Heat a non-stick ridged griddle pan over a high heat until smoking hot. Meanwhile, spray the tuna steaks all over with Fry Light and season well. Place on the griddle and cook for 2–3 minutes on each side, or until seared but still a little pink in the middle. Cut into bite-sized chunks and keep warm.

2. Arrange the lettuce, tomatoes, olives and green beans in a shallow salad bowl. Dot the eggs over the salad and season well, then scatter the tuna pieces on top. Just before serving, pour over the dressing and toss to combine.

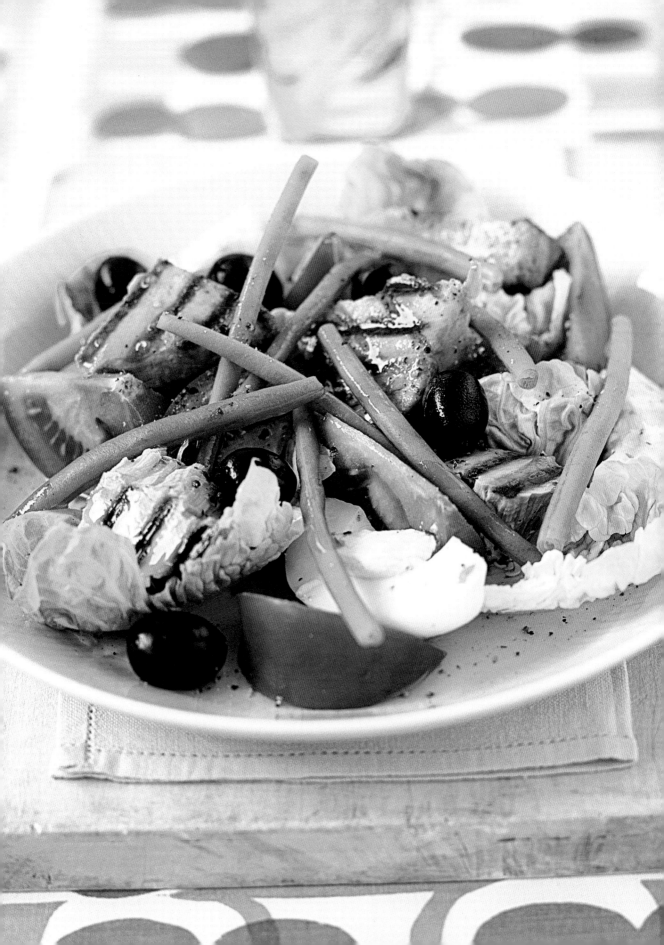

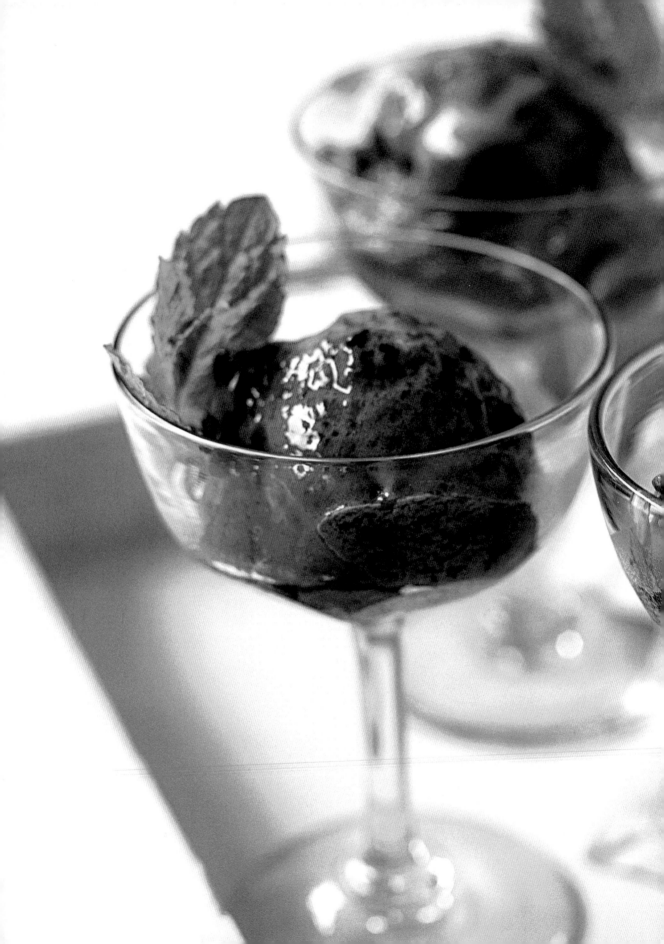

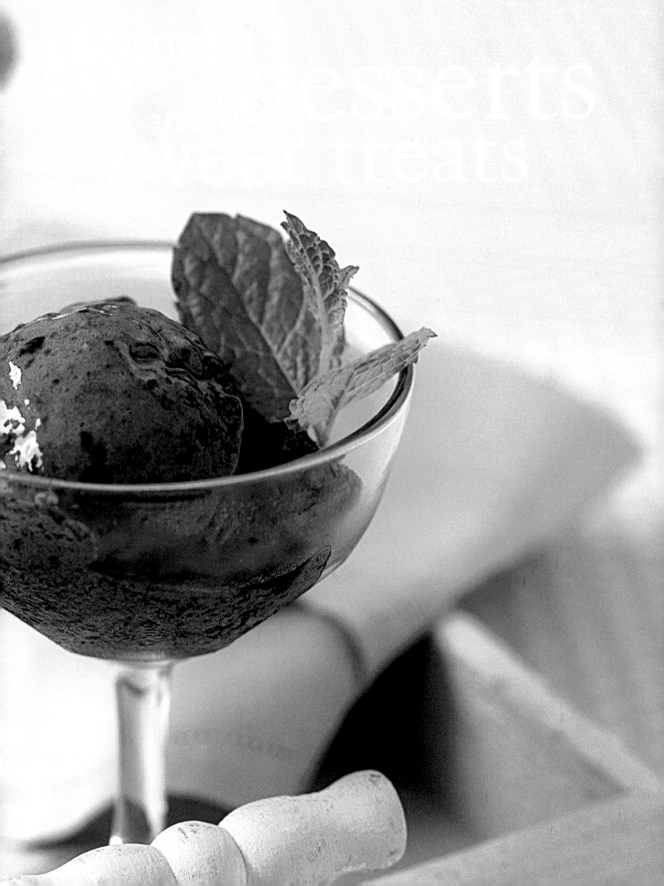

lemon
meringue pie

Everyone loves lemon meringue pie: the marshmallowy topping is a wonderful contrast to the crisp pastry case and tangy citrus filling. No wonder it's a favourite!

SERVES 8

WORTH THE EFFORT

Syns per serving
Original: 8
Green: 8

Preparation time 15–20 minutes, plus chilling
Cooking time about 30 minutes

1 tbsp flour, for dusting
250g/9oz shortcrust pastry
juice and finely grated zest of 3 lemons
600ml/22fl oz water
4 egg yolks
2 x 12g sachets sugar-free lemon jelly crystals
1 x 12g sachet powdered gelatine
10 tbsp artificial sweetener
2 egg whites

1. Preheat the oven to 180°C/Gas 4. Dust a clean work surface with flour, roll out the pastry on it and use to line a deep 18cm/7in non-stick, loose-bottomed tart tin. Line the pastry case with non-stick baking parchment, fill with baking beans and bake for 20 minutes. Remove the beans and parchment and bake for a further 5–6 minutes, or until the pastry is lightly golden and crisp. Set aside to cool in the tin.

2. Put the lemon juice and zest in a saucepan with the water and egg yolks. Place over a gentle heat and whisk constantly until the mixture starts to thicken (take care that the eggs don't curdle). Remove from the heat and whisk in the jelly crystals, gelatine and 5 tablespoons of the sweetener until thoroughly combined. Set aside to cool. When cool, spoon the mixture into the baked pastry case, cover and chill for 24 hours, or until set.

3. Just before serving, preheat the grill until hot. Whisk the egg whites until stiff and gradually fold in the remaining sweetener. Spoon this mixture evenly over the chilled lemon base, ruffle the top with a fork and grill for 1–2 minutes, until lightly golden on top. Serve immediately.

apple tart

Here's a neat idea – apple tart that includes custard within the pastry case. The luscious combination will keep you coming back for more.

SERVES 4 ⓥ

WORTH THE EFFORT

Syns per serving
Original: 8½
Green: 8½

Preparation time 5 minutes
Cooking time 30 minutes

1 tbsp flour, for dusting

110g/4oz shortcrust pastry

6 tbsp low fat custard

1 red apple, peeled, cored and very thinly sliced

2 tsp ground cinnamon

To serve

1 tsp icing sugar

1. Preheat the oven to 190°C/Gas 5. Dust a clean work surface with flour, roll out the pastry on it and use to line an 18cm/7in tart tin. Line the pastry case with non-stick baking parchment and baking beans, and bake for 10–12 minutes. Remove the beans and parchment and bake for a further 5–6 minutes, or until the pastry is lightly golden and crisp. Remove from the oven and allow to cool in the tin.

2. Spoon the custard into the pastry case and top with the apple slices. Sprinkle with the cinnamon and return to the oven for 10–12 minutes. Dust lightly with icing sugar before serving.

rice pudding

This slow-cooked rice pudding flavoured with vanilla is the ultimate comfort food – rich and creamy and well worth waiting for.

SERVES 4 ⓥ

WORTH THE EFFORT

Syns per serving

Green: 1½

Original: 8

Preparation time 15 minutes

Cooking time 1½–1¾ hours, plus resting

Fry Light

150g/5oz short grain pudding rice

400ml/14fl oz skimmed milk

400ml/14fl oz water

8–10 tbsp artificial sweetener

1 vanilla pod

1. Preheat the oven to 150°C/Gas 2. Spray a 1.5 litre/2½ pint ovenproof dish with Fry Light.

2. Rinse the rice under running cold water, drain and place in the prepared dish.

3. Place the milk, water and sweetener in a medium saucepan. Scrape in the seeds from the vanilla pod. Heat gently until almost simmering, then pour over the rice, stirring well.

4. Cook in the oven for 1½ hours, stirring after the first 30 minutes. If the pudding still seems very runny at the end of the cooking time, return it to the oven, checking every 10 minutes, until it is loosely creamy. (The cooking time will vary, depending on the type and depth of dish used.) When the pudding is golden brown on top and has a soft, creamy texture, remove from the oven and allow to rest for 10 minutes before serving.

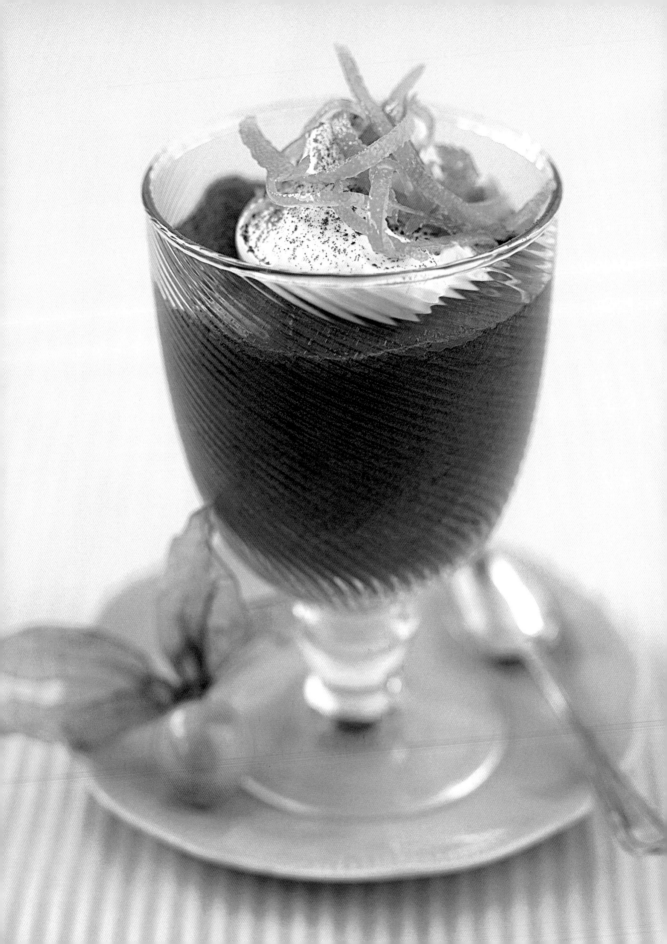

classic chocolate mousse

As this recipe contains uncooked eggs, it's not suitable for pregnant woman, toddlers and the elderly – which is a great pity as it tastes terrific!

SERVES 4 Ⓥ ❋
WORTH THE EFFORT
Syns per serving
Original: 6½
Green: 6½

Preparation time 35 minutes plus chilling

75g/3oz dark chocolate
3 medium eggs, separated
3–4 tbsp artificial sweetener
1–2 tsp finely grated orange zest
2 tbsp brandy

For the garnish
1 orange
200ml/7fl oz water
2 tbsp artificial sweetener

To serve
very low fat natural fromage frais mixed with artificial sweetener to taste
1 tsp cocoa powder

1. Break the chocolate into small pieces and place in a large, heatproof bowl. Sit the bowl over a pan of gently simmering water to melt the chocolate. Remove from the heat and allow to cool slightly at room temperature.

2. Meanwhile, whisk the egg whites in a large bowl until stiff, but not too dry.

3. In a separate bowl whisk the egg yolks, sweetener, orange zest and brandy, then spoon into the melted chocolate, mixing well.

4. Using a metal spoon, fold the egg whites into the chocolate mixture until well combined. Divide between 4 individual ramekins or dessert glasses and chill for 3–4 hours, or until set.

5. Meanwhile, make the garnish. Carefully remove long, thin strips of zest from the orange. Place in a saucepan with the water and sweetener. Bring to the boil, reduce the heat and simmer for 7–10 minutes, or until most of the liquid has evaporated. Remove the caramelised zest from the pan and leave to cool on non-stick baking parchment.

6. Before serving, top each mousse with a spoonful of the sweetened fromage frais, lightly dust with cocoa powder and garnish with the caramelised zest.

eton mess

This classic no-cook dessert should be enjoyed in the height of the summer, when English strawberries are at their best and full of sweetness.

SERVES 4

EXTRA EASY

Syns per serving
Original: 3½
Green: 3½

Preparation time 10 minutes

400g/14oz strawberries

2 x 200g pots Müllerlight strawberry yogurt

400g/14oz very low fat natural fromage frais

1 tbsp artificial sweetener

4 meringue nests, roughly crushed

To serve
whole strawberries

1. Roughly chop the strawberries, place half of them in a blender and purée until smooth. Transfer to a bowl with the yogurt and mix well.

2. Place the remaining chopped strawberries in a bowl, add the fromage frais and sweetener and stir to combine. Add to the purée mixture and swirl through to give a marbled effect. Fold in the crushed meringue and spoon this mixture into 4 chilled dessert glasses. Serve immediately, garnished with a few whole strawberries.

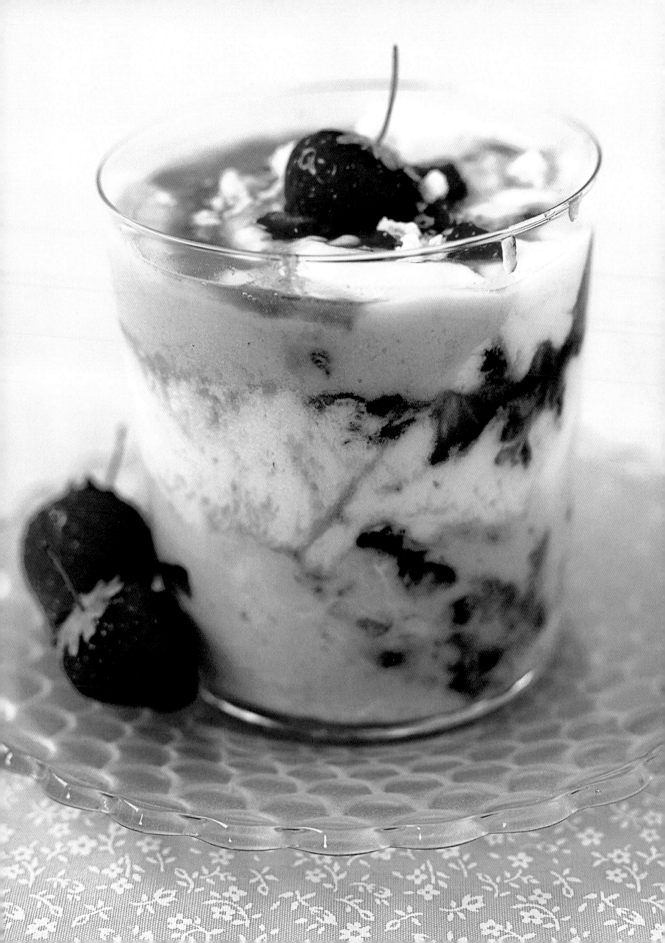

lemon syllabub

This delectable dessert is great for entertaining as it can be prepared the night before and chilled until ready to serve.

SERVES 4

EXTRA EASY

Syns per serving
Original: Free
Green: Free

Preparation time 10 minutes
plus chilling

300g/11oz very low fat natural fromage frais

200g/7oz quark

1 x 200g Müllerlight vanilla yogurt

finely grated zest of 1 small lemon

2–3 drops vanilla extract

3–4 tbsp artificial sweetener, or to taste

To serve
finely shredded lemon zest (optional)

1. Whisk together the fromage frais, quark, yogurt, lemon zest, vanilla extract and sweetener. Divide the mixture between 4 chilled dessert glasses and refrigerate for 2–3 hours, or overnight if time permits.

2. Just before serving top each glass with the shredded lemon zest, if using.

mixed berry brûlée

This is a fantastic summer treat, but it can be made at any time of year by using frozen berries: just defrost them thoroughly before proceeding with the recipe.

SERVES 4 ⓥ

EASY

Syns per serving
Original: 2
Green: 2

Preparation time 15 minutes
plus macerating

400g/14oz mixed berries
(raspberries, blackberries,
blueberries)
2 tbsp artificial sweetener
400g/14oz very low fat natural
fromage frais
8 tsp caster sugar

1. Place the berries in a bowl with the sweetener. Mix and set aside to macerate for 30 minutes.

2. Spoon the berry mixture into 4 glass ramekins and top with the fromage frais. Sprinkle 2 teaspoons of caster sugar over each one and use a kitchen blowtorch to caramelise the top. Alternatively, place the ramekins under a hot grill for 2–3 minutes. Serve immediately.

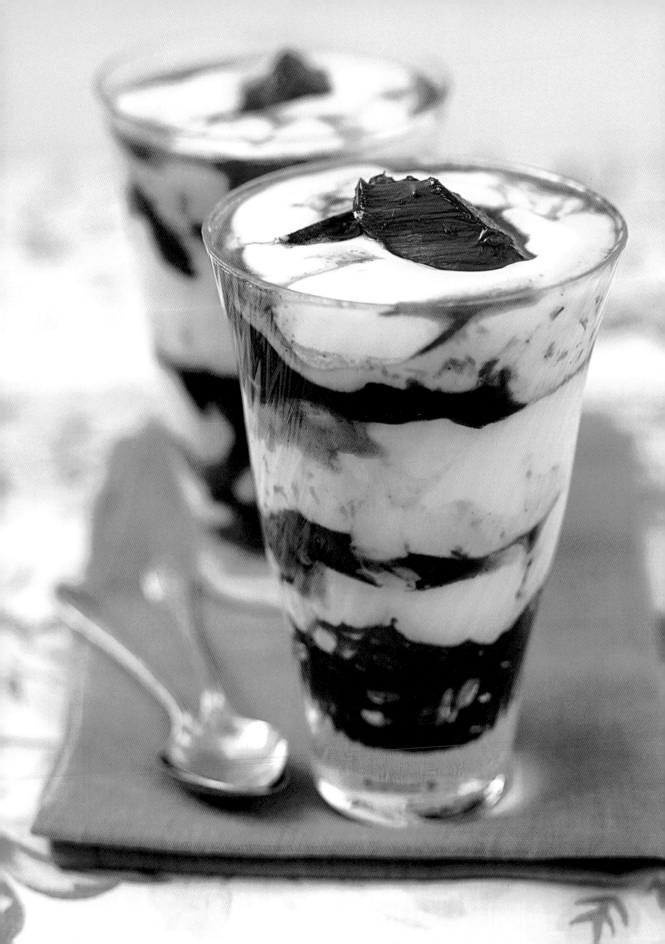

rhubarb fool

Traditional fool recipes generally include lots of whipped cream, but ours uses low fat custard. The result is a delicious healthy option that will have people clamouring for more.

SERVES 4 ⓥ

EASY

Syns per serving
Original: 4½
Green: 4½

Preparation time 10 minutes
Cooking time 20–25 minutes
plus chilling

600g/1lb 6oz rhubarb, cut into chunks
6–8 tbsp artificial sweetener
2 tsp ground ginger
1 vanilla pod, split in half lengthways
400g/14oz low fat custard

To serve
100g/3½oz very low fat natural fromage frais

1. Preheat the oven to 180°C/Gas 4. Mix the rhubarb, sweetener, ginger and vanilla in an ovenproof baking dish and place in the oven for 20–25 minutes, until the rhubarb is soft. Transfer the mixture to a large bowl, discarding the vanilla pod, and set aside to cool.

2. When cool, layer the rhubarb and custard in 4 tall dessert glasses and refrigerate for 2–3 hours. Top with the fromage frais before serving.

crêpes suzette

Flavoured with orange zest and juice, these thin dessert pancakes make a yummy and impressive finish to a meal.

MAKES 4 ⓥ

WORTH THE EFFORT

Syns per serving
Original: 7½
Green: 7½

Preparation time 20 minutes
Cooking time about 15–20 minutes

150g/5oz plain flour
3 tbsp artificial sweetener
a pinch of salt
2 large eggs, beaten
250ml/9fl oz skimmed milk
2–3 drops vanilla extract
1 tbsp orange juice
1 tbsp finely grated orange zest
Fry Light

For the sauce
juice of 2 oranges
2–3 tbsp artificial sweetener

To serve
very low fat natural fromage frais mixed with artificial sweetener to taste

1. Start by making the sauce. Place the ingredients in a small saucepan over a gentle heat and stir until the sweetener has dissolved. Remove from the heat and set aside.

2. Sift the flour, sweetener and salt into a bowl. Mix in the eggs, milk, vanilla extract, orange juice and zest, whisking until smooth.

3. Spray a 15cm/6in frying pan with Fry Light and place over a high heat. When hot, pour in about a quarter of the batter, tilting the pan to spread it evenly. Cook for 1–2 minutes, or until the pancake is lightly browned underneath. Flip over and cook the other side for 1–2 minutes. Remove, fold into quarters and keep warm while you cook the remaining crêpes.

4. To serve, place the folded crêpes on warmed serving plates, drizzle with the orange sauce and serve with a spoonful of the sweetened fromage frais.

apple and cinnamon crumbles

Here's a treat for all the family. The soft apple contrasts beautifully with the crunchy crumble, and the aroma of cinnamon is irresistible.

SERVES 4 Ⓥ ❄

EASY

Syns per serving
Original: 10
Green: 10

Preparation time 15 minutes
Cooking time 15–20 minutes

800g/1lb 12oz cooking apples

1–2 tbsp artificial sweetener

50g/2oz wholemeal self-raising flour

1 tsp ground cinnamon

¼ tsp ground allspice

50g/2oz low fat spread, suitable for baking (such as Anchor Lighter Spreadable)

4 tsp soft brown sugar

1. Preheat the oven to 190°C/Gas 5. Quarter the apples, discard the cores and chop into bite-sized chunks. Divide between 4 individual baking dishes, add 1 tablespoon of water to each dish and sprinkle over the sweetener. Set aside.

2. Sift the flour, cinnamon and allspice into a mixing bowl, add the low fat spread and rub together, using your fingertips, until the mixture resembles breadcrumbs. Spoon over the apples and top with the sugar.

3. Place the dishes on a baking sheet and bake for 15–20 minutes, or until the apple is bubbling and the top is crisp and golden. Serve immediately.

steamed ginger puddings

Perfect for a cold day, these warm steamed puddings are rich with the flavours of spice and ginger. Serve with low fat custard for an indulgent ending to a meal.

SERVES 4 ⓥ

WORTH THE EFFORT

Syns per serving
Original: 6½
Green: 6½

Preparation time 15 minutes
Cooking time 20–25 minutes

Fry Light
4 tbsp reduced sugar apricot jam
2 eggs, separated
28g/1oz golden caster sugar
4 tbsp artificial sweetener
75g/3oz self-raising flour
3 tsp ground ginger
½ tsp ground allspice
1 tbsp finely chopped stem ginger

To serve
low fat custard (optional)

1. Preheat the oven to 200°C/Gas 6. Spray 4 individual pudding basins with Fry Light and place in a deep roasting tin. Spoon 1 tablespoon of jam into each of the basins.

2. Whisk the egg yolks with the sugar and sweetener until pale and fluffy. Sift in the flour, ground ginger and allspice and mix well.

3. Whisk the egg whites until softly peaked, then fold into the yolk mixture with the stem ginger. Spoon into the prepared basins, cover with non-stick baking parchment and foil and pour boiling water into the roasting tin to come halfway up the sides of the basins. Place in the oven and steam for 20–25 minutes, or until the puddings are just firm and springy to the touch.

4. Put a plate over each basin and invert to turn out the puddings. Serve with low fat custard if desired (1½ Syns per 2 tbsp).

chocolate and orange
bread pudding

Here's a fantastic variation on an old favourite. The longer you leave the pudding, the firmer it becomes, because the custard sets inside the bread.

SERVES 6

WORTH THE EFFORT

Syns per serving
Original: 5½
Green: 5½

Preparation time 20 minutes
Cooking time 30 minutes plus standing

8 slices Nimble white bread

4 tbsp reduced sugar marmalade

4 large eggs

350g/12oz very low fat natural fromage frais

25g/1oz cocoa powder

1 tsp finely grated orange zest

5–6 tbsp artificial sweetener, or to taste

To serve

6 tbsp very low fat natural fromage frais mixed with artificial sweetener to taste

15g/½oz dark chocolate

orange zest

1. Preheat the oven to 180°C/Gas 4. Spread 4 slices of bread with the marmalade, then top with the remaining slices to make 4 sandwiches. Cut into quarters and arrange in a small, ovenproof baking dish, overlapping them to fit.

2. Place the eggs and fromage frais in a bowl and beat together. Sift in the cocoa and mix until well combined. Stir in the orange zest and add sweetener to taste.

3. Spoon the cocoa mixture over the sandwiches to cover them completely, making sure it sinks between them as well.

4. Stand the dish in a roasting tin and pour in boiling water to come halfway up the side of the dish. Bake for 25–30 minutes, until just set. Remove from the tin of water and leave to stand for 10 minutes.

5. Divide the pudding between 4 bowls and place a dollop of sweetened fromage frais on each. Grate the chocolate over the top, sprinkle with orange zest and serve straight away.

individual
summer puddings

Soft fruits, particularly berries, are among the great delights of summer food. Their colour, texture and flavour can be enjoyed to the max in these classic summer puddings.

SERVES 4 Ⓥ

WORTH THE EFFORT

Syns per serving

Original: 7½

Green: 7½

Preparation time 30 minutes plus overnight chilling

Cooking time 8–10 minutes

10 medium slices slightly stale, good-quality white bread, crusts removed

225g/8oz blueberries

225g/8oz blackberries

225g/8oz raspberries

100ml/3½fl oz water

10–12 tbsp artificial sweetener

To serve

very low fat natural fromage frais (optional)

1. Line 4 individual pudding basins with cling film, then use the bread slices to line the basins, trimming them to fit and reserving some slices for the 'lids'.

2. Place the fruit and water in a saucepan. Sprinkle over the sweetener and bring to a simmer over a low heat, stirring occasionally, for 8–10 minutes. Set aside to cool completely.

3. Using a slotted spoon, fill the prepared bowls with the cooked fruit. Cover each with a lid of the reserved bread and trim neatly around the edges. Cover with cling film, then place the bowls on a tray and put a small plate on top of each pudding. Sit a can of baked beans on each plate as a weight and refrigerate for 24 hours, or up to 3 days if time permits.

4. To serve, remove the weights and small plates. Place a shallow dish or serving plate over each basin and carefully invert the pudding. Carefully peel off the cling film and serve with fromage frais, if desired.

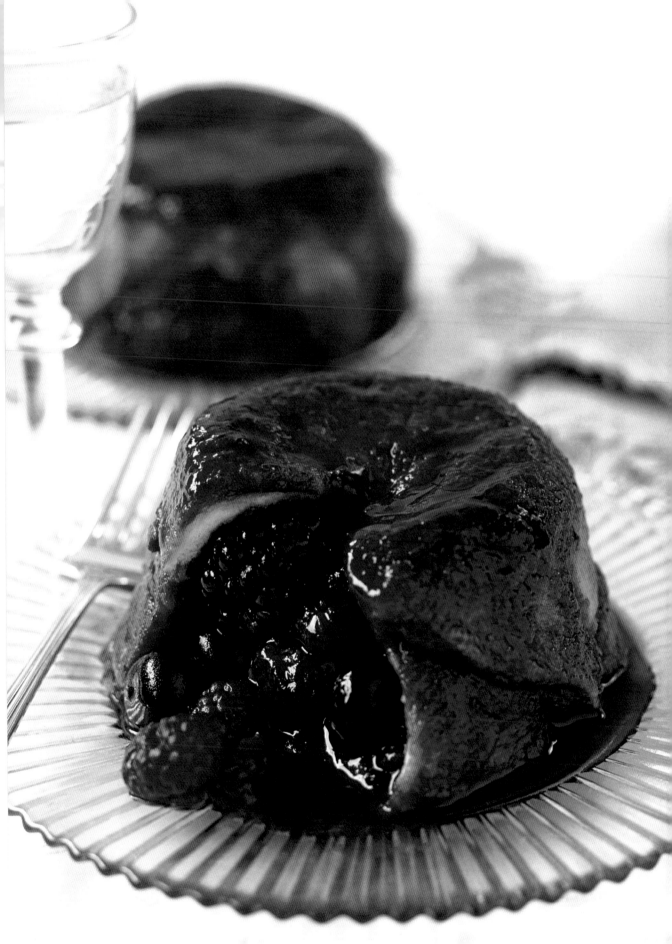

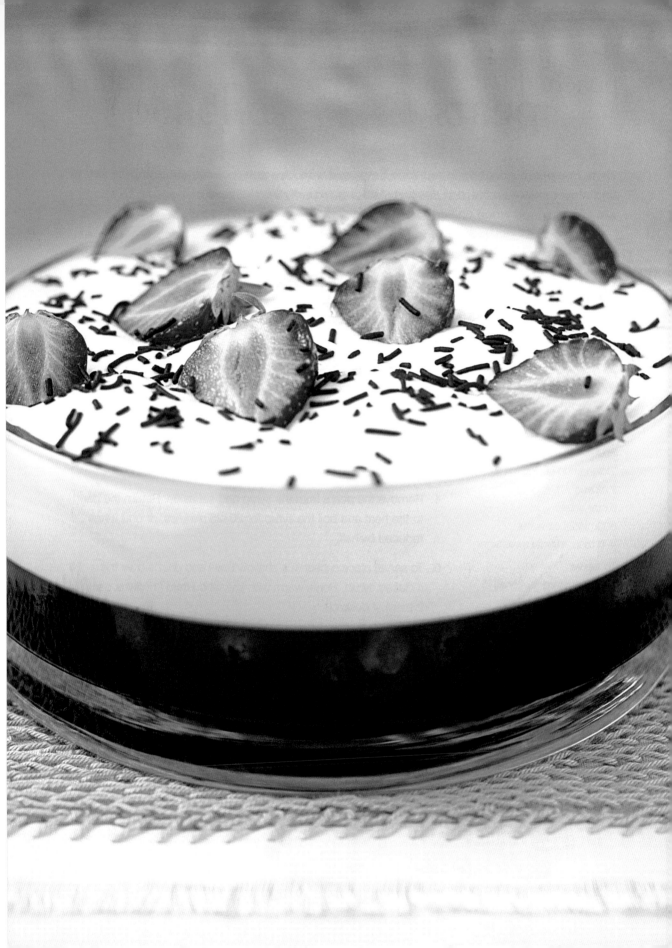

sherry trifle

This low-Syn delicious trifle combines jelly, berries, low fat custard and a creamy topping made with fromage frais and quark.

SERVES 8
WORTH THE EFFORT
Syns per serving
Original: 3
Green: 3

Preparation time 25 minutes plus chilling

1 x 12g sachet sugar-free raspberry jelly crystals

400ml/14fl oz boiling water

2 tbsp sherry

450g/1lb mixed berries (blackberries, blueberries and raspberries)

1 tbsp artificial sweetener, plus exra to taste

500g/1lb 2oz low fat custard

250g/9oz quark

250g/9oz very low fat natural fromage frais

To serve
strawberries, halved
1 tsp chocolate vermicelli

1. Make up the jelly with the boiling water and allow to cool. Stir in the sherry.

2. Place the berries in a medium-sized trifle bowl, sprinkle with the sweetener and mix well.

3. Pour the cooled jelly mixture over the berries, then cover and chill for 3–4 hours, or until set.

4. Pour the custard over the set jelly mixture.

5. Make up the topping by whisking together the quark, fromage frais and sweetener to taste until smooth. Spoon the mixture over the custard, then chill for 2–3 hours before serving topped with the strawberries and sprinkled with chocolate vermicelli.

carrot cake

Moist carrot cake is really delicious, and so simple to prepare. Here we've made it extra indulgent by adding a cream cheese-style topping.

SERVES 8 ⓥ

WORTH THE EFFORT

Syns per serving

Original: 2½

Green: 2½

Preparation time 10 minutes

Cooking time 40–45 minutes

100g/3½oz plain flour

1 tsp bicarbonate of soda

2 eggs, lightly beaten

150ml/5fl oz skimmed milk

2 tsp ground cinnamon

2 tsp ground allspice

2 tsp ground ginger

3 large carrots, peeled and coarsely grated

6–8 tbsp artificial sweetener

2 tsp grated orange zest

For the topping

200g/7oz quark

vanilla extract

artificial sweetener, to taste

1. Preheat the oven to 180°C/Gas 4. Line a medium non-stick loaf tin with baking parchment.

2. Place the flour and bicarbonate of soda in a bowl and add the eggs, milk, spices, carrots, sweetener and orange zest. Mix well, then spoon into the prepared tin. Bake in the oven for 40–45 minutes, until golden and cooked through. Remove from the oven and leave to cool in the tin for about 10 minutes, then turn out onto a rack and allow to cool completely.

3. Meanwhile, make the topping. Place the quark in a bowl and whisk in a few drops of vanilla extract and sweetener to taste. Chill until needed.

4. Once the cake has cooled, spread the quark mixture over the top and serve cut into slices.

lemon drizzle cake

Teatime becomes a special occasion when it's accompanied by something home-baked. This moist and zesty cake is a real treat.

SERVES 10 Ⓥ

WORTH THE EFFORT

Syns per serving
Original: 4
Green: 4

Preparation time 25 minutes
Cooking time 30–35 minutes

4 eggs, separated
50g/2oz caster sugar
5 tbsp artificial sweetener
150g/5oz self-raising flour
1 tsp baking powder
2 tbsp finely grated lemon zest
1 tsp icing sugar, to dust

For the drizzle
long strips of zest from
2 lemons
juice of 2 lemons
1 tbsp arrowroot
4 tbsp artificial sweetener
60ml/2fl oz water

1. Preheat the oven to 190°C/Gas 5. Line a 22cm/9in cake tin with non-stick baking parchment.

2. Place the egg yolks, caster sugar, sweetener, flour, baking powder and lemon zest in a bowl and whisk until thick and pale.

3. In a separate bowl whisk the egg whites until softly peaked, then fold into the yolk mixture. Spoon into the prepared tin and place in the oven for 25–30 minutes, or until the cake has risen and is firm to the touch. Leave to cool.

4. Meanwhile, place all the drizzle ingredients in a small saucepan and bring to the boil, whisking constantly. When the liquid starts to thicken, remove from the heat and leave to cool. Drizzle the sauce over the cake and allow to set.

5. Once the sauce has set, dust the cake with icing sugar and serve cut into wedges.

chocolate and apricot brownies

Rich and delectable, brownies must be one of the best-ever American inventions. Here's our version, with nuggets of apricot for extra texture.

MAKES 24 Ⓥ ❋

EASY

Syns per brownie
Original: 4
Green: 4

Preparation time 15 minutes
Cooking time 18–20 minutes

110g/4oz low fat spread, suitable for baking (such as Anchor Lighter Spreadable)

8 tbsp drinking chocolate powder

4 tbsp artificial sweetener

60g/2½oz caster sugar

3 eggs

100g/4oz self-raising flour

1 tsp baking powder

250g/9oz dried apricots, chopped

1 tsp vanilla extract

1. Preheat the oven to 180°C/Gas 4 and line a 30 x 20cm/12 x 8in baking tin with non-stick baking parchment.

2. Melt the low fat spread in a saucepan, remove from the heat and stir in the drinking chocolate, sweetener and sugar. Add the eggs and whisk until combined.

3. Sift in the flour and baking powder and stir well. Mix in the apricots and vanilla extract, then pour into the prepared tin and bake for 18–20 minutes, until just set (it will firm as it cools). While still warm, turn out onto a board and cut into 24 portions.

black forest roulade

The combination of cherries, chocolate sponge and sweetened 'cream' has been a restaurant favourite for decades. Now you can make our version of what many consider to be the perfect dessert.

SERVES 8 Ⓥ
WORTH THE EFFORT

Syns per serving
Original: 4½
Green: 4½

Preparation time 10 minutes
Cooking time 15–18 minutes
plus chilling

6 large eggs, separated
100g/3½oz caster sugar
8 tbsp artificial sweetener
50g/2oz cocoa powder
100g/3½oz very low fat natural fromage frais
200g/7oz quark
170g/6oz canned pitted cherries in juice, drained and chopped

To serve
1 tsp icing sugar
1 tsp cocoa powder

1. Preheat the oven to 180°C/Gas 4. Line a 30 x 20cm/12 x 8in swiss roll tin with non-stick baking parchment.

2. Whisk together the egg yolks, sugar and 5 tablespoons of the sweetener until thick and pale. Sift in the cocoa, then fold together using a metal spoon.

3. Whisk the egg whites in a separate bowl until just stiff and fold into the yolk mixture. Spoon into the prepared tin and bake for 15–18 minutes, or until set and springy to the touch. Leave to cool in the tin.

4. Place a large sheet of baking parchment on a work surface. Turn the sponge onto it, then peel away its lining paper.

5. Whisk the fromage frais with the quark and the remaining 3 tablespoons of sweetener and spread carefully over the sponge. Scatter the cherries over the surface.

6. Lift one end of the parchment and roll up the sponge (don't worry if it cracks). Place the roulade seam-side down on a platter and chill for 1–2 hours.

7. Before serving, mix together the icing sugar and cocoa, and dust over the surface of the roulade. Serve cut into thick slices.

banoffee pie

Great for hassle-free entertaining, this delicious banana-topped pie is flavoured with toffee and vanilla, and for extra indulgence is drizzled with melted chocolate.

SERVES 8

WORTH THE EFFORT

Syns per serving
Original: 4½
Green: 4½

Preparation time 30 minutes
Cooking time 15 minutes plus chilling

10 reduced fat digestive biscuits, finely crushed

3 medium egg whites

2 x 12g sachets powdered gelatine

75ml/3fl oz boiling water

250g/9oz quark

3 x 200g pots Müllerlight toffee yogurt

3–4 tbsp artificial sweetener

1 tsp vanilla extract

2 bananas

To serve

dark chocolate, melted (optional)

cinnamon, to dust

1. Preheat the oven to 190°C/Gas 5. Line a 20cm/8in springform cake tin with baking parchment.

2. Place the crushed biscuits in a bowl. Lightly beat 1 of the egg whites until frothy and add to the bowl. Stir well, then spoon the mixture into the prepared tin and press evenly over the bottom. Bake in the oven for 15 minutes, then set aside to cool.

3. Dissolve the gelatine in the boiling water.

4. Whisk the quark in a bowl until smooth. Stir in the yogurt, sweetener and vanilla extract.

5. Whisk the 2 remaining egg whites until stiff, then fold into the quark mixture along with the gelatine liquid. Spoon over the prepared biscuit base, smoothing the top with a palette knife, and chill for 4–5 hours, or until set.

6. Remove the pie from the tin and place on a serving plate. Slice the bananas and arrange neatly on top of the pie. Drizzle over some melted dark chocolate (1½ Syns per 1 tsp) if desired, dust with cinnamon and serve cut into wedges.

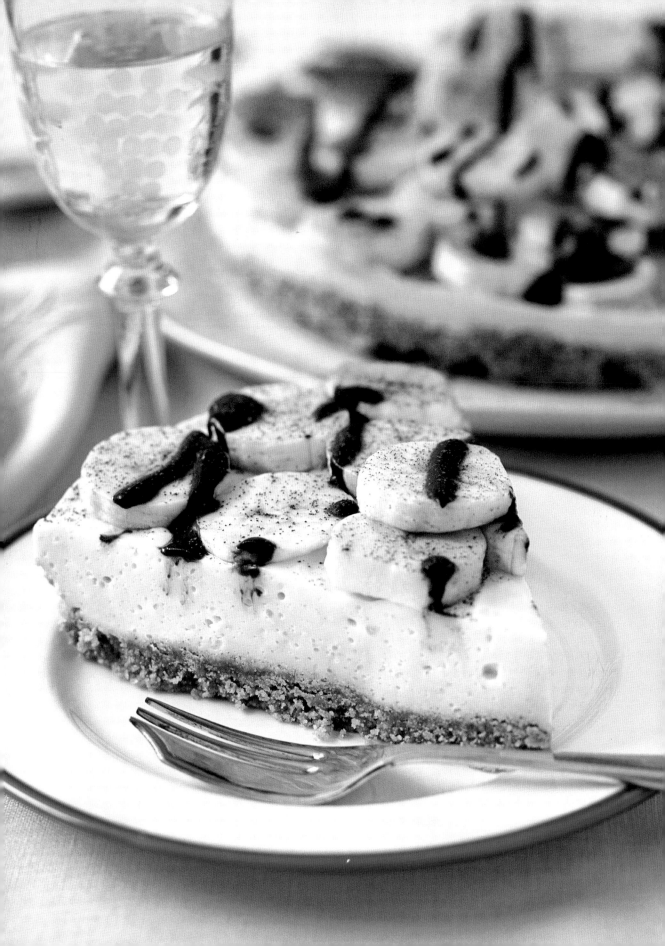

vanilla cheesecake

For an impressive summer dessert, serve this cheesecake piled with fresh summer berries and dusted with icing sugar.

SERVES 8

WORTH THE EFFORT

Syns per serving

Original: 5

Green: 5

Preparation time 25 minutes
plus chilling

8 reduced fat digestive biscuits, finely crushed

50g/2oz low fat spread, melted

1 x 12g sachet sugar-free lemon jelly crystals

150ml/5 fl oz boiling water

1 tsp powdered gelatine

2 x 200g pots Müllerlight vanilla yogurt

1–2 tsp vanilla extract

1 tbsp finely grated lemon zest

200g/7oz quark

4–5 tbsp artificial sweetener, or to taste

To serve

chopped fresh fruit of your choice

cocoa powder or icing sugar (optional)

1. Mix together the crushed biscuits and melted spread and arrange evenly in the bottom of a 20cm/8in springform cake tin. Flatten with the back of a spoon and refrigerate for 30 minutes.

2. Make up the jelly with the boiling water and stir in the gelatine. When cool, place the jelly mixture in a food processor with the yogurt, vanilla extract, lemon zest, quark and sweetener. Process until smooth, then pour over the biscuit base. Cover and refrigerate overnight or until set.

3. To serve, remove the cheesecake from the tin and place on a platter. Arrange the fresh fruit over the top and dust lightly with cocoa or icing sugar (1 Syn per 1 tsp), if using.

chocolate chip
cookies

Ideal for elevenses or a teatime treat, these cookies have all the flavour of shop-bought ones, but much less of the fat.

MAKES 18 Ⓥ
EASY
Syns per cookie
Original: 3½
Green: 3½

Preparation time about 15 minutes
Cooking time 12–15 minutes

175g/6oz self-raising flour
75g/3oz low fat spread, suitable for baking (such as Anchor Lighter Spreadable)
12 tbsp artificial sweetener
60g/2½oz chocolate chips
3 tbsp very low fat natural fromage frais
1 egg yolk

1. Preheat the oven to 180°C/Gas 4 and line a baking sheet with non-stick baking parchment.

2. Sift the flour into a bowl, add the spread and rub it in using your fingertips until the mixture resembles breadcrumbs. Sprinkle over the sweetener and mix well.

3. Stir in the chocolate chips, fromage frais and egg yolk, then knead with your hands to form a soft dough. Divide the mixture into 18 pieces and roll each one into a ball. Place the dough balls on the prepared baking sheet and flatten them into cookie shapes by pressing lightly with the back of a damp fork.

4. Bake in the oven for 12–15 minutes, or until golden. Transfer to a wire rack and cool before serving.

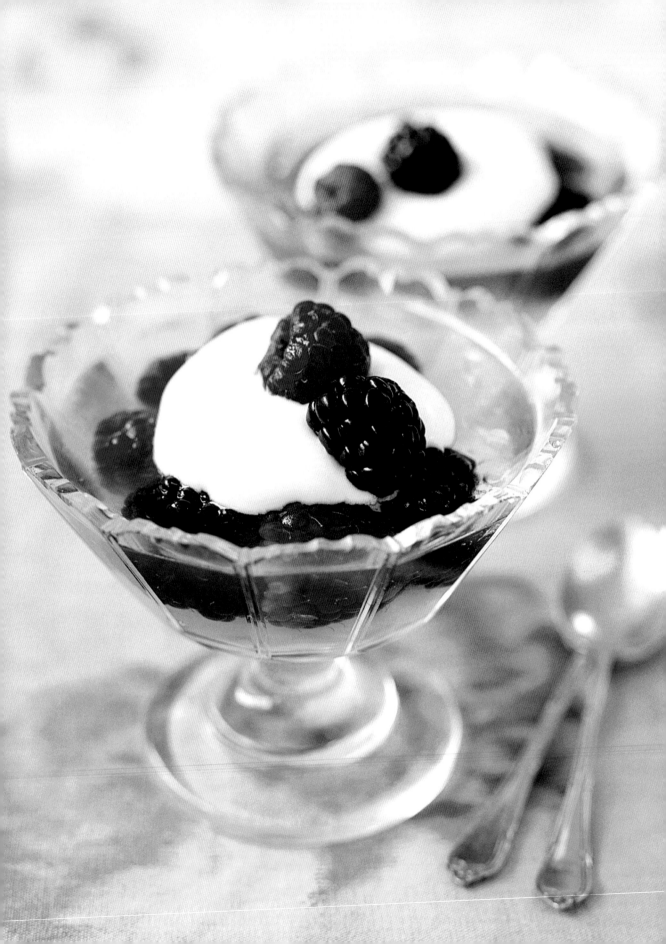

raspberry and blackberry jellies

Fruit and jelly make a great dessert for kids and adults alike. Our sophisticated version includes lots of luscious fresh berries.

SERVES 4

EASY

Syns per serving
Original: 1
Green: 1

Preparation time 10 minutes plus chilling

300g/11oz raspberries
100g/3½oz blackberries
2 x 12g sachets sugar-free lemon jelly crystals

To serve

4 tbsp very low fat natural yogurt
raspberries and blackberries

1. Divide the berries between 4 large dessert glasses. Place in the fridge to chill.

2. Make the jelly according to the packet instructions and, when cool, pour over the chilled fruit. Refrigerate for 5–6 hours, or until just set.

3. To serve, place 1 tablespoon of yogurt on top of each jelly and garnish with raspberries and blackberries.

ultimate fruit salad

Here we have a fabulous selection of fruit flavoured with a lightly spiced syrup – a simple but colourful dessert that's a great way to end a meal.

SERVES 6 ⓥ

EASY

Syns per serving
Original: ½
Green: ½

Preparation time 20 minutes
Cooking time 3–4 minutes

2 apples, cored and cut into bite-sized cubes

1 kiwi fruit, peeled and cut into bite-sized cubes

200g/7oz pineapple, cut into bite-sized cubes

¼ orange-fleshed melon, peeled, deseeded and cut into bite-sized cubes

1 banana, thickly sliced

100g/3½oz red and green seedless grapes

For the syrup

1 tbsp very finely diced stem ginger

1 tbsp runny honey

1 tbsp lemon juice

¼ tsp ground ginger

75ml/3fl oz water

1–2 tsp artificial sweetener (optional)

To serve

mint leaves

very low fat natural fromage frais (optional)

1. Start by making the syrup. Place the stem ginger, honey, lemon juice, ground ginger and water in a small saucepan, and add the sweetener, if using. Stir well and bring to the boil. Remove from the heat and allow to stand for 5–6 minutes.

2. Place the fruit in a serving bowl and mix well.

3. Pour the syrup over the fruit salad, mix well and serve garnished with mint leaves. Accompany with fromage frais, if desired.

creamy
mango sorbet

As a refreshing treat on a hot summer's day, or a light dessert after a rich meal, you can't go wrong with this delicious sorbet.

SERVES 4 ❋
WORTH THE EFFORT
Syns per serving
Original: 2½
Green: 2½

Preparation time 10 minutes
plus freezing

350g/12oz mango, peeled and stoned
2–3 tbsp artificial sweetener
200g pot Müllerlight vanilla yogurt

To serve
mango slices

1. Place the mango flesh in a food processor with the sweetener and yogurt. Blend until smooth, then pour into a freezerproof container. Freeze for 2–3 hours, or until the sides and base of the sorbet have started to set but the centre is still liquid. Beat the mixture with a fork, then return to the freezer for 4–5 hours, beating every 30 minutes to break up the ice crystals.

2. When the sorbet is finally solid, transfer to the fridge for 10–15 minutes to soften slightly before serving. Scoop into bowls and garnish with the mango slices.

ice cream

A great freezer standby for last-minute entertaining, ice cream is really easy to make, and the four varieties given here are packed with flavour. Note that the strawberry, chocolate and vanilla recipes contain uncooked eggs, so should not be served to those in vulnerable health groups.

strawberry ice cream

SERVES 4 ❋

EASY

Syns per serving
Original: 1½
Green: 1½

Preparation time 20 minutes
plus freezing

450g/1lb strawberries
6 tbsp artificial sweetener
1–2 tsp lemon juice
2 x 200g pots Müllerlight strawberry yogurt
1 egg white, lightly beaten until frothy

1. Place the strawberries in a food processor with the sweetener and blend until smooth. Using the back of a spoon, push this mixture through a fine sieve into a bowl, discarding the seeds.

2. Mix the lemon juice, yogurt and beaten egg white into the strawberry mixture, then pour into a shallow, freezerproof container. Cover and freeze for about 1½–2 hours.

3. Place the ice cream in the food processor and blend until smooth. Return to the shallow container and freeze for 4–5 hours, or until solid. Before serving, allow the ice cream to soften at room temperature for 10–15 minutes.

chocolate ice cream

SERVES 4 ❋

EASY

Syns per serving
Original: 1½
Green: 1½

Preparation time 25 minutes
plus freezing

3 x 11g sachets Cadbury Highlights hot chocolate drink
2 x 200g pots Müllerlight vanilla yogurt
2 egg whites

1. Empty the Highlights sachets into a bowl, add 6 tablespoons of boiling water and mix until smooth. Set aside to cool. When cool, whisk in the yogurt.

2. Beat the egg whites until frothy and fold into the yogurt mixture. Transfer to a shallow, freezerproof container, cover and freeze for 3–4 hours, or until firm. Before serving, allow the ice cream to soften at room temperature for 10–15 minutes.

vanilla ice cream

SERVES 4 ❋

EASY

Syns per serving
Original: Free
Green: Free

Preparation time 20 minutes
plus freezing

3 eggs, separated
8–10 tbsp artificial sweetener
1 tsp vanilla extract
350g/12oz Müllerlight vanilla
yogurt

1. Beat the egg yolks with the sweetener and vanilla extract until pale and thick.

2. In a separate bowl, beat the egg whites until just stiff, then fold into the yolk mixture. Add the yogurt and mix well.

3. Transfer the mixture to a shallow, freezerproof container, then cover and freeze, stirring every 30 minutes, or until the ice cream is solid. Before serving, allow to soften at room temperature for 10–15 minutes.

mint ice cream

SERVES 4 ❋

EASY

Syns per serving
Original: Free
Green: Free

Preparation time about 15
minutes plus freezing

400g/14oz very low fat natural
fromage frais
1 tsp green food colouring
1 tsp peppermint extract
1 tbsp artificial sweetener

1. Place the fromage frais in a mixing bowl. Add the remaining ingredients and whisk until light and fluffy.

2. Pour the mixture into a freezerproof container, cover and freeze for about 4 hours, stirring every 30 minutes to break up any ice crystals.

3. Before serving, allow the ice cream to soften at room temperature for 10–15 minutes.

summer berry sorbet

Desserts don't come any easier – or quicker – than this one. Using frozen berries means that it's an 'instant' sorbet and needs no further freezing.

SERVES 4

EXTRA EASY

Syns per serving
Original: 1½
Green: 1½

Preparation time 5 minutes

500g/1lb 2oz frozen summer berries

300g/11oz very low fat fruit yogurt

2 tbsp artificial sweetener

1. Place all the ingredients in a food processor and blend briefly. Scrape the mixture from the sides and blend again.

2. Spoon the sorbet into chilled dessert glasses or bowls and serve immediately

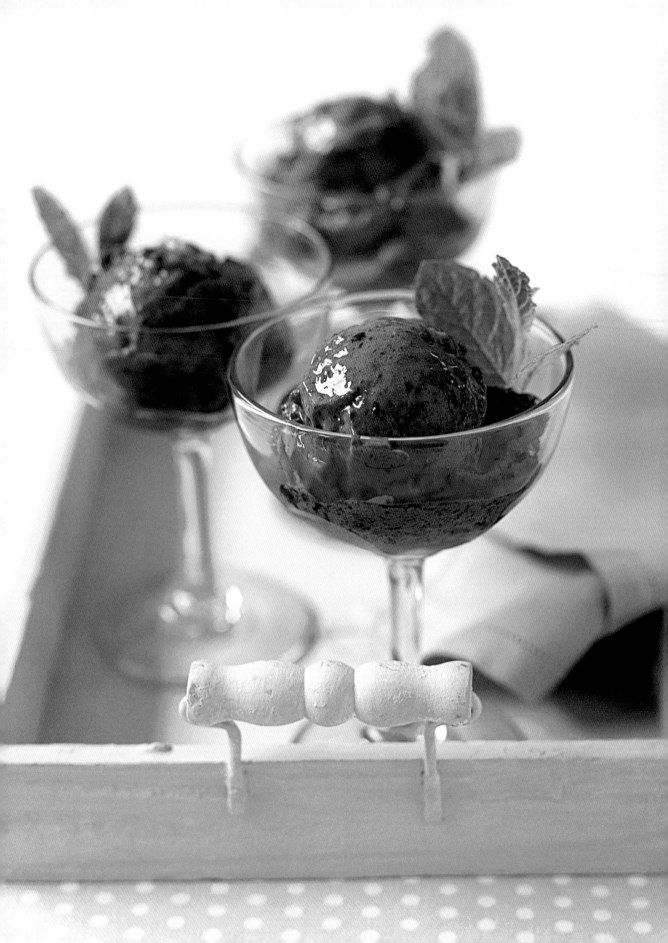

the changing shape
of britain

Forty years ago, when the first Slimming World groups opened in Derbyshire, few people could have foreseen just how great a problem obesity would become. While excess weight was a big issue for the individuals concerned, it wasn't seen as a topic of national importance. Today, with 20 per cent of men and 23 per cent of women obese, and a further 43 per cent of men and 33 per cent of women overweight, our 'obesity epidemic' is rarely out of the headlines. As well as having a dramatic impact on the health and happiness of over half the population, obesity costs billions of pounds to the NHS and to employers in lost working days, while every year over 34,000 deaths in the UK can be attributed to it.

How has this 'epidemic' come about? A government report in 2007 referred to our 'obesogenic' environment – acknowledging that changes in society have made the energy gap (the difference between the energy we take in as food and the energy we use in everyday life) grow steadily in the past few decades. There are more opportunities than ever before to make high-fat food choices, with a fast-food takeaway or coffee shop on every corner, supermarkets bursting with ready meals and low-cost alcohol and eating out becoming an everyday occurrence. Hugely increased car use, the rise of sedentary office jobs over manual jobs, Internet shopping and home computers, meanwhile, have meant that our activity levels are lower than they've ever been.

Over the next few pages, we'll look in more detail at how our changing lifestyles have had a dramatic impact on our weight and our health, and how our environment has made it harder than ever to maintain a healthy weight. The message is clear: there has never been a greater need for an effective way to lose weight and to maintain a healthy weight in the long term. So 40 years on, it's not surprising that Slimming World's combination of healthy eating, motivating group support and lifestyle-based activity is in greater demand – from individuals looking for personal help and from the NHS searching for national solutions – than ever before.

food
fashions

The 1973 'Martians' commercial for Smash instant potato ('They peel them with their metal knives, boil them for 20 of their minutes – then they smash them all to bits!') remains one of Britain's all-time favourite ads. And in some

ways the humble spud sums up the most fundamental change in our diet over the past 40 years. In 1974 the average consumption per person was around 1kg (2¼lb) of fresh potatoes per week; by 2006 this figure had

The Smash advert's aliens persuaded us that instant mashed potato was a reality, not just a futuristic dream.

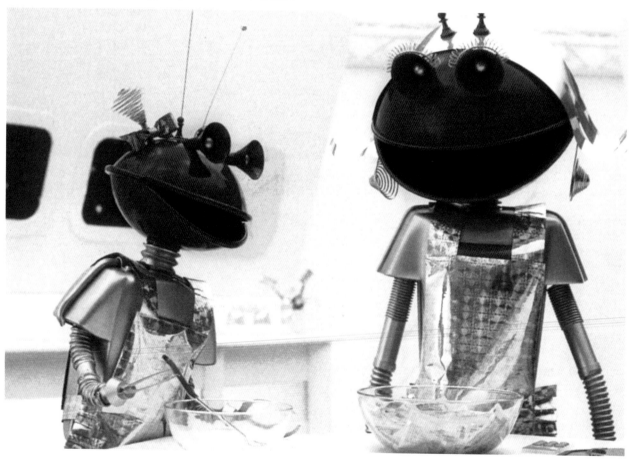

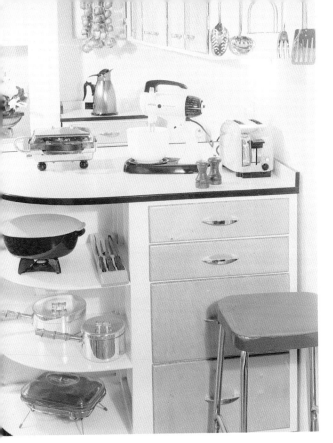

The 1960s' kitchen had many 'mod cons', but it had only a tiny fridge, reflecting the fact that most food was freshly made on a daily basis.

bag of pre-cut chips, whereas preparing fresh potatoes actually uses up calories (even more if you walk to the shop and carry them home).

Meanwhile, developments in technology also meant that the relative price of food began to fall; in 1971 we spent around 20 per cent of our household budget on food, but by 2006 food accounted for just under 10 per cent. As processing costs came down, foods that had once been seen as occasional treats, such as fizzy drinks, ice cream and crisps, became much more affordable.

And, thanks to longer shop-opening hours and the growing trend for commuting by car and eating on the move, buying food anywhere and everywhere became much easier too. The explosion in out-of-home eating and snacking has had a major influence on our diet in the past 40 years: in 2006 the average household spent £53.40 per week on food to eat at home, and £31.90 on food and drink in restaurants, pubs and takeaways.

> *Since the 1970s, the time we spend preparing the main meal of the day has dropped from an hour to around 20 minutes.*

In fact, if a Slimming World member from 1969 could have time-travelled 40 years into the future, she'd probably have wondered how 21st-century slimmers coped, constantly surrounded by opportunities to eat, and in portion sizes much bigger than she would be used to.

In 1969 takeaway choices were largely limited to fish and chips (or maybe a Wimpy

halved, but the amount of processed potatoes eaten had more than doubled.

This and many other crucial developments can be traced to the early 1970s. By then most households had a fridge and often a freezer, microwave ovens were starting to appear, and supermarkets were springing up everywhere. In 1960 convenience foods represented about a fifth of the food we ate; by 1970 this had risen to a quarter, and it's continued rising. The growth in convenience foods certainly saved time and energy: the amount of time spent preparing the main meal of the day has dropped from an hour to around 20 minutes.

Labour-saving products, such as ready meals and other pre-prepared foods, have allowed calorie-burning opportunities to slip out of our day: it takes hardly any energy to open a

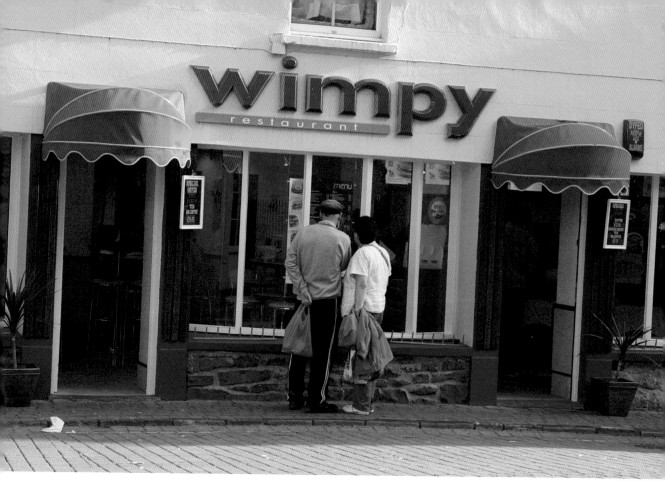

Britain's first taste of American fast food came courtesy of Wimpy bars, which sold hamburgers named after Popeye's friend J. Wellington Wimpy.

burger) as the boom in Indian, Chinese, pizza and burger restaurants did not start until the mid-1970s. A shopping trip to town might have included a cup of tea (40 calories) and a small

> *We now spend nearly as much of our weekly budget eating out in restaurants as we do eating at home.*

scone (150 calories), while in 2009 our choices would be more likely to include a large latte coffee (a whopping 265 calories) and a giant muffin (600 calories). Having a coffee shop on

every corner isn't always a good thing for slimmers!

Our 1969 slimmer would also be astonished by the sheer variety of foods on sale, as immigration, overseas travel and cheaper imports have transformed our food horizons in the past 40 years. In 1974 olive oil was mainly on sale for medicinal purposes, and rice was used in puddings, not curries. Today chicken tikka masala is regularly voted our 'national dish', and supermarkets are full of exotic ingredients, from lemongrass to linguine.

It's not just trends in food that have changed – our drinking habits have dramatically altered too. Our alcohol intake has gone up from 5.5 litres (9½ pints) per head in 1969 to 9 litres

(16 pints) per head in 2006, with much of the increase accounted for by wine. Forty per cent of men and a third of women admit to exceeding the healthy drinking limit on at least one occasion a week, and alcohol-related deaths have more than doubled since 1991.

But it's not all bad news for slimmers. Our overall diet has actually changed for the better in some ways. Our average daily calorie count is lower than it was in 1974 – we now consume around 2,300 on average compared to just over 2,500 calories 35 years ago. This is mainly because we eat less fat than we used to, with many more low fat dairy products and leaner meat on sale. We also eat more vegetables and fruit than before, although our tastes have changed: we eat fewer apples and pears, and more grapes, bananas and soft fruit. As a result, our daily fruit and veg total has risen from three to nearly four portions on average. However, we still eat more fat, sugar and salt than the government recommends for health, much of it in processed foods, where it's harder to recognise, despite the current drive for clearer and more prominent food labelling.

And that, of course, makes Slimming World's clear, straightforward path through the food maze even more valuable to 21st-century slimmers. By focusing on simple, everyday ingredients, which are highly satisfying and packed with nutritional goodness but low in fat, Slimming World helps its members make the most of today's abundant food choices and still lose weight.

then and now

then: lentils, wholemeal bread and muesli were 'hippie food'.

now: pulses and wholegrains are super-healthy foods.

then: a cupboard full of tins and a very small fridge.

now: hardly any tins and a huge fridge-freezer.

then: a glass of wine at Christmas.

now: bottles of wine on the weekly shopping list.

then: eating Italian, Indian or Chinese foods only in restaurants.

now: 'pinging' Italian, Indian or Chinese in the microwave every week.

then: olive oil from the chemist for earache.

now: extra virgin olive oil from the supermarket for salads.

then: around 20 per cent of the average household budget went on food.

now: we spend just under 10 per cent of our budget on food.

then: on average we drank 5.5 litres (11½ pints) of alcohol in a year.

now: the average has risen to 9 litres (19 pints) per year.

how we work, how we live

In 1966 the comedian Tony Hancock advised us all to 'Go to work on an egg' in one of the most memorable advertising slogans of the past 40 years. And in those days a lot more people needed to start the day with a hearty breakfast: in 1971 nearly a third of men and just

Eggs were a favourite way to start the day in the 1960s and '70s, but as jobs became more sedentary in later decades, many people stopped eating breakfast at all.

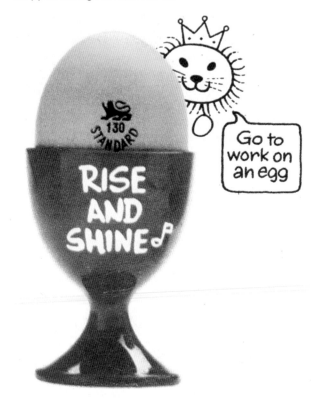

Go to work on an egg

under a fifth of women worked in the traditional industries of manufacturing, mining and farming. By 2006 this had fallen to 17 per cent of men and just 6 per cent of women.

Over the past 40 years, more and more of us have moved into jobs that involve sitting on our bottom all day rather than doing any physical labour. While this has made working conditions a lot better for many of us, it's not surprising more of us than ever are struggling to control our weight.

Changes in our working life have had a big impact on family life too. In 1971 just over half

In 1971 just over half of women of working age had a job outside the home, while today around 70 per cent of women do.

of women of working age had a job outside the home, while today seven out of ten women do.

Britain's transformation from a manufacturing to a service economy has been good for our health in many ways – especially for men, who are less at risk of occupational diseases and accidents. However, there have been downsides too. Working hours for British families are still some of the longest in Europe, with more women in particular now working longer hours. Research indicates that this in itself may be contributing to our national weight problem, as countries with longer working hours tend to have higher obesity levels.

Technology and changing work practices have also seen to it that we use less energy in our working life than ever before. Even a sedentary job in the 1960s, such as working in a typing pool, still involved hammering the

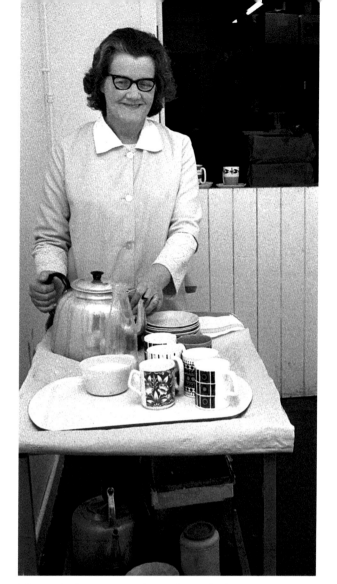

The tea lady was a regular and popular feature of the typical British office – until vending machines and coffee shops took over.

then and now

then: getting your wages in a brown envelope every week.

now: having your salary paid into your bank account every month.

then: walking around the whole building to circulate a memo.

now: sending a memo to everyone with the click of a mouse

then: work stopped whenever the building was closed.

now: work can be accessed 24/7 online

then: the tea trolley and canteen

now: breakfast from Starbucks and lunch from Subway.

then: going to the travel agent in your lunch hour to book your holiday.

now: booking your holiday online in your lunch hour.

keys of a manual typewriter, running off document copies by hand, and fetching and carrying papers and messages through the building. Today it takes almost no calories to send an email compared to walking across the floor to talk to a colleague, and almost no energy to travel three floors in the lift rather than walk up the stairs.

In 1969 banking was available only during office hours, while shops closed at 6 p.m. and were shut all day Sunday. Even the BBC told us when to go to bed by playing the national anthem and switching off the signal! In 2009 we enjoy 24-hour service seven days a week, and working patterns have been adapted to suit, with more people than ever employed on split shifts, nights and weekends. This in turn has had a big impact on family life, as parents aim to juggle work and childcare. The good news is that this has led to more equality between the sexes (some women might find this hard to believe, but men's share of housework and childcare has doubled on average in the past 30 years). However, eating healthily and exercising can also be a challenge for people who work shifts; in a recent survey, 80 per cent of women who worked shifts said they had put on weight through not being able to plan their meals.

These new ways of working have brought many advantages – more flexibility, more opportunities for women, and a freedom of choice we wouldn't have dreamed of in the 1960s – as well as, in general, more affluence. They've also created new challenges.

Thanks to its flexible approach and emphasis on freedom of choice, Slimming World is uniquely placed to help 21st-century slimmers have the best of all worlds!

CHANGING LIFESTYLES

When Slimming World launched 40 years ago exercise and fitness weren't really part of the vocabulary. Most people kept fit through their active lifestyle at work and at home, so going to a gym to work out simply wasn't necessary. Men who wanted more muscles would secretly buy a 'Bullworker' machine and use it at home, while for women who wanted to slim, the emphasis was on strict calorie-counting rather than burning more energy through exercise

(though you could buy vibrating belts that were supposed to pummel the fat away).

This all changed in the 1980s, when gym membership became popular as part of the 'work hard, play hard' culture. Films such as *Flashdance* and *Fame* made working out look sexy, and in 1982 along came Jane Fonda with her aerobics videos, prompting a whole generation of women to wriggle into leotards, tights and woolly legwarmers.

On average we walk 63 fewer miles per year in our daily life than we did in 1975/6 – the equivalent of around 6,300 calories or 1kg (2¼lb) of fat gained without changing our diet in any way.

Since then the fitness industry in the UK has grown and grown, and is now valued at more than £3 billion, with more than one in ten of us having gym membership (though research also shows that a significant number of those gym passes never get used after the first week). Yet we haven't seen corresponding increases in the nation's fitness; in fact, by many measures we are less active than previous generations who didn't have the access to leisure facilities that we have today. One in three adults surveyed in 2007 said they had done no active sport in the past 12 months. And, amazingly, on average we walk 63 fewer miles per year in our daily life than we did in 1975/6 – that's the equivalent of around 6,300 calories or 1kg (2¼lb) of fat gained, without changing our diet in any way at all.

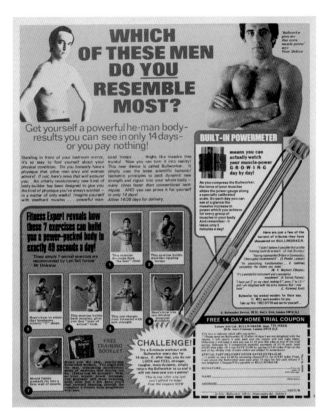
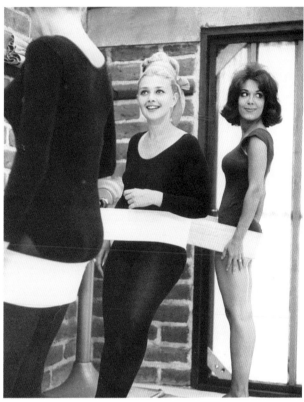

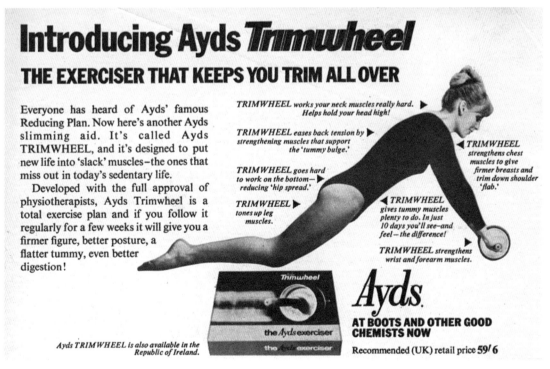

Introducing Ayds *Trimwheel*

THE EXERCISER THAT KEEPS YOU TRIM ALL OVER

Everyone has heard of Ayds' famous Reducing Plan. Now here's another Ayds slimming aid. It's called Ayds TRIMWHEEL, and it's designed to put new life into 'slack' muscles—the ones that miss out in today's sedentary life.

Developed with the full approval of physiotherapists, Ayds Trimwheel is a total exercise plan and if you follow it regularly for a few weeks it will give you a firmer figure, better posture, a flatter tummy, even better digestion!

TRIMWHEEL works your neck muscles really hard. Helps hold your head high!

TRIMWHEEL eases back tension by strengthening muscles that support the 'tummy bulge.'

TRIMWHEEL goes hard to work on the bottom—reducing 'hip spread.'

TRIMWHEEL tones up leg muscles.

TRIMWHEEL strengthens chest muscles to give firmer breasts and trim down shoulder 'flab.'

TRIMWHEEL gives tummy muscles plenty to do. In just 10 days you'll see—and feel—the difference!

TRIMWHEEL strengthens wrist and forearm muscles.

Ayds TRIMWHEEL is also available in the Republic of Ireland.

the Ayds exerciser

Ayds.

AT BOOTS AND OTHER GOOD CHEMISTS NOW

Recommended (UK) retail price 59/6

Over the last four decades there have been all manner of weird and wonderful ways to keep fit and lose weight. Here are just a few of them.

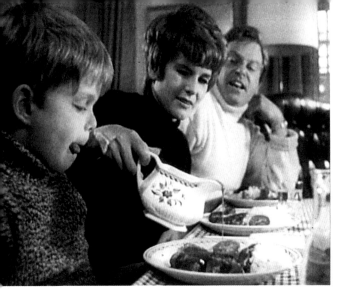

The Oxo ad featured a typical British family enjoying a home-cooked meal. Eating habits have now changed so much that Oxo have abandoned this approach.

So if we're not out there walking, what are we doing instead? The answer is probably: sitting down! In 1969 we were already a nation of telly addicts; 91 per cent of homes had a TV, although there were only three channels: BBC1, ITV and the five-year-old BBC2.

The 1970s saw the introduction of the first TV remote control – depriving us of another opportunity to burn a few calories each evening as we got up to change channels – and the first video recorders, so TV watching was no longer limited to broadcasting hours. Going to the cinema gradually became less popular than renting films to view at home.

One of the biggest revolutions of the past 40 years, however, has been the rise of home-based entertainment beyond the TV. We now spend nine times more on communication and eight times more on recreation every year than we did in 1971 – mainly on home computing, video and electronic games, music equipment and mobile phones. While the amount of power used in home cooking has dropped by a third in 35 years, the amount used on electrical appliances such as computers and TVs has more than doubled in the same period.

A recent survey estimated that young men spend around 12 hours a week on average playing video and computer games, while a 2006 survey estimated that children spend an average of 588 hours a year watching TV – that's 24 days! Add to that the facts that parents' safety concerns mean that fewer children these days are allowed to play outside unsupervised, and over half of children now travel to school by car, even if they live within walking distance, and it's not surprising that childhood obesity is one of our fastest-growing problems.

'Social networking' is the latest trend to keep us even more closely tied to our computer screens. Forty years ago teenagers kept in touch with their friends by going to each others' houses. Now friendships are carried out on the Internet via sites such as Facebook and MySpace instead.

The amount of power used in home cooking has dropped by a third in 35 years, while the amount used on computers and TVs has doubled.

But the TV and computer aren't the only life-style changes contributing to our obesity levels. In 1971 just over half of households had the regular use of a car. By 2006 the number of licensed drivers had risen from 20 million to 34 million, and one in four households have two cars or more.

Labour-saving devices in the home have freed people (mainly, it has to be said, women)

then and now

then: Mum cooking dinner ready for when Dad came home.

now: Dad cooking dinner while Mum works late.

then: sitting around the table eating Sunday lunch.

now: going out shopping and then for pizzas on a Sunday.

then: making children come in from playing outside.

now: making children leave their computers to play outside.

then: staying in to watch *Coronation Street*.

now: going out, then catching *Coronation Street* later on Sky+.

then: talking to your best friend on the phone in the hall.

now: talking to lots of friends at once on Facebook.

spending more and more time online: according to 2008 figures, 32.5 million people have Internet access, and the average broadband user spends 16 hours a week online. In the last few years the chance to shop online and have everything delivered has taken the hassle out of the weekly supermarket trip for thousands of families, although it has also removed the opportunity to burn a couple of hundred calories pushing a trolley for an hour, compared to the tiny amount of energy it takes to push a computer mouse around a desk.

Very few of us would want to turn the clock back to the '70s, as today's lifestyle offers so much variety and richness. Finding ways to combine it with enough activity to keep us fit for life is the challenge we all face – and it's one that Slimming World's Body Magic programme (see page 18 for further information) was designed to meet.

Although many women might disagree, there's no doubt that modern men do more household chores than previous generations.

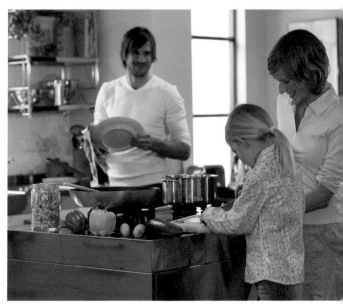

a lot of the drudgery of housework. The energy required to manage the 1960s' household was far higher than today, when most households have vacuum cleaners, washing-machines and tumble-driers, and fridge-freezers big enough to store a month's shopping at a time.

Overall we spend far less time on daily chores than we did in the 1970s, but we are

fats and figures

In 1969 Margaret Miles-Bramwell's liberating and enjoyable approach to losing weight was like an oasis of common sense for would-be slimmers who were in the grip of a calorie-counted, restrictive diet – and that's still the case today.

Nimble bread was one of the best-known 'slimming foods' of the 1960s and '70s.

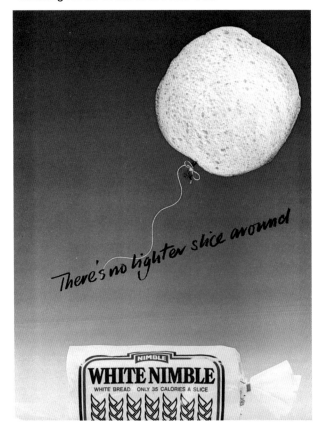

There's no lighter slice around

NIMBLE
WHITE NIMBLE
WHITE BREAD ONLY 35 CALORIES A SLICE

Over the past 40 years, calorie-restricting diets have come in all kinds of weird and wonderful variations, and even now hardly a week goes by without another daft idea hitting the headlines. Remember, for instance, the Grapefruit Diet (eat a whole, raw grapefruit before each meal), the Egg Diet (eat up to nine a day) and the Cabbage Soup Diet (eat…well, you get the idea)?

There have been numerous theories about various food groups, such as fat: the idea that eating fat is satisfying and therefore helps you lose weight was part of the reasoning behind the Atkins Diet, which was first launched in the 1970s and reappeared for a short while only a few years ago. Sugar also became the villain of the piece after a 1972 book called *Pure, White and Deadly* blamed it for all our ills. In 1982 Audrey Eyton's influential *F-Plan Diet* put carbohydrates back on the menu for slimmers. From the 1970s onwards the pharmaceutical and food industries began to realise that there was a growing market for slimming products, and brought science to bear on diets based on very low-calorie meal replacements. In the same decade we were treated to slimmers' biscuits, diet meals in a can, special drinks and sweets (remember Diet Ayds?) to help you suppress your appetite, and slimmers' bread – all with the emphasis firmly on calorie control rather than health. Later came diet drinks made with artificial sweeteners, and a huge range of 'lite', lower-calorie versions of high-fat favourite foods.

Fortunately, Slimming World members have never had to swallow lemon juice for breakfast, survive on soup, or eat nothing but bananas and boiled eggs. While most members do find that Food Optimising works beautifully for them and they reach their target weight quickly, they are also made aware from the start that there is no such thing as a 'quick fix'. What Slimming World offers is a lasting solution, which involves making permanent lifestyle changes.

THE RISE OF OBESITY

Although women – and some men, though fewer than today – worried about their weight in 1969 (not surprising when Twiggy was the fashion icon of the day), the 'obesity crisis' was still many years away. Collecting statistics about the number of overweight people was not a priority, and although we gained weight as a nation during the 1970s, only 6 per cent of men and 8 per cent of women were obese by 1980.

Since then, the number of overweight and obese people in the UK has risen steadily. There are now 24 million people who are overweight or obese – 63 per cent of men and 56 per cent of women – and in more recent

> *In 1980 just 6 per cent of women were obese; now an alarming 56 per cent are either overweight or obese.*

years the figures have been climbing faster than ever: in the decade ending in 2004, the proportion of obese men rose by over 50 per cent, and of obese women by 36 per cent.

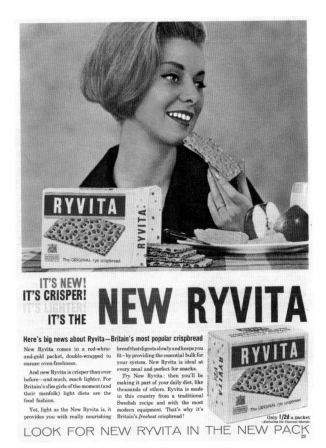

First produced in 1930, Ryvita is still going strong, although these days it shares the market with a multitude of other 'healthier' foods.

Even more worryingly for our future health as a nation, three in ten boys and girls aged 2–15 are classed as obese or overweight.

As we have already seen, the effects of our increasingly 'obesogenic' environment are proving extremely hard for the majority of people in the UK to resist. As a result, obesity is now being officially described as presenting as big a threat to public health as climate change and smoking.

Helping patients to manage their weight is now higher on the medical profession's agenda than it has ever been. The first prescription-only weight-loss drugs became available ten years ago, and GPs now hand out more than a million prescriptions for them each year, even though

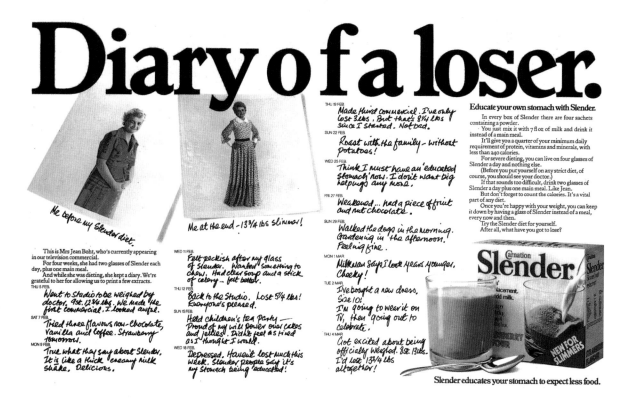

Meal-replacement drinks have been around for decades – but why use them when you can eat anything you want with Slimming World and still lose weight?

they have side-effects and still require lifestyle changes. Weight-loss surgery is now officially approved as a treatment for people whose weight is causing them severe health problems.

Since the 1990s, scientists have made several important discoveries in genetics and neurology that may yet produce more effective weight-loss treatments. There is a great deal of research into how hormones affect our appetite, and whether some people are more genetically predisposed to put on weight than others. However, no one has yet come up with a way to short-circuit our highly efficient metabolism, evolved over thousands of generations, which, unfortunately, makes our body very good at storing fat and very slow at burning it off.

In the meantime, the Slimming World approach, which is to help raise members' awareness of their own food pitfalls and to make lifestyle changes as easy and enjoyable as possible, is increasingly being recognised as a practical and powerful solution, and is widely used by the National Health Service through the many 'Slimming World on Referral' schemes that Slimming World has pioneered in the past few years.

There's no such thing as a 'quick fix'. Instead Slimming World offers its members a lasting solution.

It has been forecast that the obesity crisis could take 30 years to turn around. With 40 years' experience of helping hundreds of thousands of slimmers solve their own personal obesity crisis, Slimming World could not be better placed to face the challenges ahead.

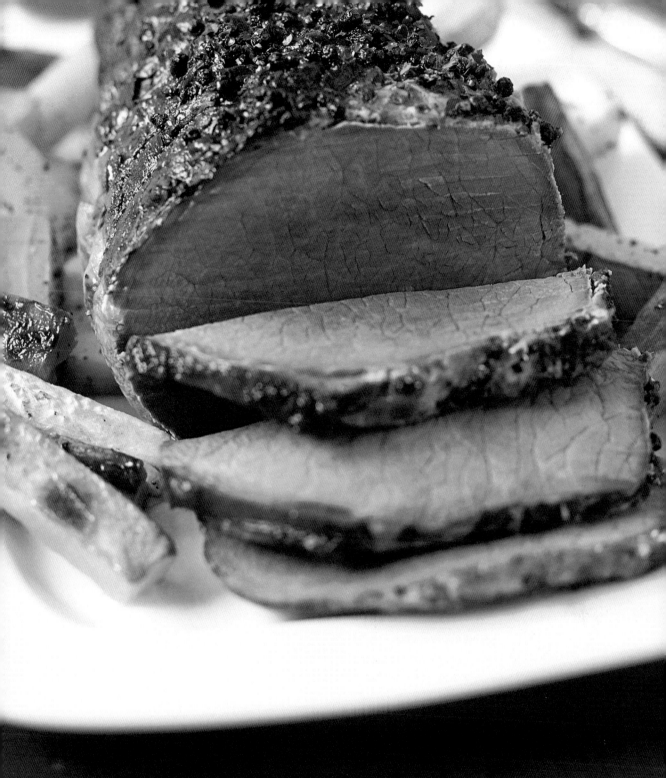

index